Core Exercises for Seniors Over 60

Guided Daily Exercises Designed to Build Strength, Improve Balance and Stability, and Increase Energy for Active Aging Adults

By: Mason Hayes

Core Exercises for Seniors Over 60: Guided Daily Exercises Designed to Build Strength, Improve Balance and Stability, and Increase Energy for Active Aging Adults

Table of Contents

Introduction

The abdominals and supporting musculature are one of the more essential subsystems and groups of muscles in the body. Though every muscle and system in the body is important, these sets of muscles act as the nucleus or center point of our movement and deserve a little more attention. These muscles are constantly working to maintain posture, remove stress from the spine, allow us to bend and twist easily, and move our upper and lower extremities with power and strength! Think about this region of your body like a corset or weight belt. The abdominal muscles wrap around our entire torso and spine, helping protect it during every movement. Having active and engaged muscles help us move more efficiently and safely. But what really makes up our core? We generally know that this includes our "abs," but it's really a multitude of muscles, including the *transverse abdominis, rectus abdominis, external and internal obliques, as well as upper body muscles such as your lats and lower body muscles including your glutes.*

Loss of muscle mass and strength is a natural part of aging, but you can keep this phenomenon at bay or slow it down to a great degree. The age-old adage "use it or lose it" perfectly describes our relationship with fitness, and it affects everyone worldwide. Building and incorporating an exercise routine into your daily life will help ensure your muscles are consistently challenged. This challenge helps our body build more muscle and encourages adaptation. These aspects of exercise will keep us strong and able to move around more safely and with confidence for many years to come.

According to the CDC (2023) about 36 million falls occur among individuals 65 years of age and older each year in the United States. That's about one in four people over 65! Roughly 32,000 deaths result from these falls, and one in five falls causes a broken bone. Women tend to fall more often than men, accounting for about 3/4 of all hip fractures. Aside from broken bones, falls can also cause traumatic brain injuries (TBIs), which come with their own set of complications. In terms of financial costs, as of 2015 (CDC), medical costs associated with falls exceed $50 billion a year, with Medicare and Medicaid paying for about 75% of these. So, what can be done to reduce your chances of falling? There are a few things that you can do to prevent falls and maintain your freedom, including getting your eyes checked regularly, managing your medication at yearly check-ups or when you feel there's a need, making your home and areas you frequent safer, AND strength training regularly making sure to incorporate postural stability and abdominal training into that program.

Studies show that regular core and postural strength training can decrease the number of falls and improve overall balance and stability, exponentially increasing quality of life. For example, a 2013 systematic review shows that core strength training, in particular, increased strength by 30% and balance and stability by 23%. A 2012 randomized controlled study looked at the impact of a 9-week progressive core instability training program on overall fitness and found that individuals improved their strength and increased spinal stability by 11%. This better allowed them to bend forward, backward, and side-to-side. Results from a Fitness, Arthritis, and Seniors

Trial (FAST) study done in 2015 showed that long-term (at least 18 months) strength training programs, in addition to regular walking, resulted in improved stability and less postural sway that can often contribute to falls.

Benefits of a strong core:

- Can better maintain activities of daily living (ADLs)
- Prolonged independence and mobility
- Better balance, coordination, and stability
- Decreased risk of falls and a better ability to get back up after a fall.
- Less likely to injure yourself overall
- Can breathe with more ease and get more air per breath
- Will remain continent for longer
- Will improve your overall health
- Can reduce pain in other areas of the body, such as joints and other muscles
- Overall, you will be able to continuously enjoy the activities you know and love for longer

In this book, we'll delve deeper into each muscle and muscle group, the most beneficial exercises, how to train and strengthen your core, and discuss how to choose the exercises that will benefit you most.

The exercises and routines provided will be easy to follow and require little to no equipment. You will also find modifications to many of these popular exercises and learn how each activity supports other muscles in the body, how those other muscles contribute to core strength, and how to turn almost any workout into an exercise that includes the abdominals and other postural stabilizers.

For most, their priorities lie in simply being able to do the things we enjoy with our loved ones. In addition, maintaining independence and mobility are also hugely important. Our muscle strength and their function lie at the heart of these priorities. They let our body move purposefully and offer protection if and when accidents happen. Without a solid and stable core, you may decline physically and mentally faster than necessary. The good news? YOU have the ability to make sure that doesn't happen. When you combine your knowledge and dedication with consistency, the information and tools included in this book will guide you toward progress and success!

CHAPTER 1 – The Core and it's Function

What is the core?
Our core plays a stabilization role in the body every single time we move. If the movement doesn't begin in the core it passes through the muscles that comprise it and more specifically, will work to carry or direct the load (or action) around the spine as opposed to through it. The main stabilizer (or postural stabilizers) muscles include the pelvic floor, transverse abdominis (TVA), internal obliques, multifidus, and diaphragm. Other muscles (the global movers) that help to move our body while stabilizing, include the rectus abdominis, erector spinae, external obliques, and quadratus lumborum. Also included are upper body muscles, such as the latissimus dorsi and trapezius, along with some lower body muscles such as the glutes and hamstrings. These muscles all function as one to assist us in performing many tasks such as the examples below.

For example;

Putting on a seatbelt
When you reach across your body to grab a seat belt, your abs and spinal stabilizer muscles (multifidus and erector spinae) stiffen so the spine can twist safely and your arm can move freely. You may also push into the seat with your leg (gluteus maximus and glute medius) to boost yourself up to make the grab a little easier on your arm. You grab the seat belt, and to begin drawing it across your body, those abdominals and spinal muscles remain stiff so you can twist back safely and click the seatbelt into place.

Getting out of a chair
As you scoot forward and prepare to get up from a chair, your spinal stabilizer muscles (multifidus and erector spinae) stiffen, and your internal and external obliques engage, allowing you to move your hips forward while keeping your spine in alignment. If you brace yourself on the arm of the chair or table and lean forward to stand, your rectus abdominis helps pull you forward, and your latissimus dorsi, and trapezius engage, helping to hold your body weight while your legs make their way underneath you. Then your gluteus maximus, gluteus medius, and hamstrings take over, allowing you to stand.

These are examples of how your core works with your body to let your arms and legs work more efficiently during everyday functions. Your abs are active during many benign and simple movements, allowing you to safely stand up and sit down. Most of these activities are ones we don't think much about in the moment.

When your toe catches

Imagine you are out on a walk, and your toe catches a small sidewalk or curb crack. Initially, your whole body stiffens up, beginning at the spine in the center of your body (multifidus, erector spinae, transverse abdominis). It does this so you have the extra strength and energy to bring a leg forward to keep yourself from falling, while simultaneously protecting the spine if your trip results in a fall. However, if your core muscles are weak or out of practice your body may not be able to compensate quickly enough or be strong enough to prevent you from falling. Aside from falling, this lack of control leaves your spine vulnerable to injury.

This is an example of how a weak, unstable, or poorly trained core can lead to more serious problems from a common accident, like tripping, that happens to many of us on a daily basis.

If your core is weak, every part of your body will attempt to compensate. From your arms and legs to muscles in your back, each of these has to work that much harder and over time requires a lot of energy that could be used elsewhere. Once your energy reserves are diminished, you're at an even higher risk of falling or simply not being able to complete activities of daily living. Core exercises can help you stay mobile and independent longer. Granted you won't be working out like you're 20 years old, and loss of muscle mass is an inherent part of aging, but working on a strong, stable core will certainly help.

The next time you reach for something or go to get up from a chair, pay attention to how it feels. This body awareness will serve you in the future and keep you in tune with how well your body actually functions.

Your core musculature can be split into two main groups: stabilizers and global movers. To work properly and effectively, these muscle groups must work together in a sequential firing order (much like spark plugs for a car). The core stabilizers are muscles associated with postural control and don't move the body around very much. The global movers produce more significant body movements and must work in conjunction with the stabilizers to work properly.

If dysfunction occurs with any stabilizer muscle(s), the mobilizer(s) or global movers will be disadvantaged. If dysfunction happens with the mobilizer(s) or global movers, injury to the stabilizer(s) will most likely occur.

Additional support comes from three subsystems (groups of muscles working together) that work like a sling crossing the body diagonally, much like the diagonal wood or cable pieces on a gate door to keep it from sagging. These subsystems are the *Anterior Oblique Subsystem, Posterior Oblique Subsystem, and the Intrinsic Stabilization Subsystem*[5].

CORE STABILIZERS

Pelvic floor
- Acts like a hammock for the bladder, colon, rectum, vagina, cervix and uterus
- Maintains control of your fecal and urinary continence
- Imperative for proper urination, defecation, sexual activity, and childbirth

Transverse abdominis

- Supports your whole lumbopelvic (low back/pelvis) region
- Maintains abdominal tension (bracing)

Proper bracing achieves the best transfer of power throughout the entire body. It isn't particularly difficult to do, but it can take time to perfect.

- Increases intra-abdominal pressure that is used in forceful expiration, coughing, and defecation but also to stabilize the spine when moving around or exercising.

Internal Obliques
- Helps to stabilize the spine as we bend forward and backward
- Helps to bend the body side to side
- Helps with breathing during exhalation (works opposite the diaphragm)

Multifidus (also semispinalis and rotatores to form the transversospinalis)
- Continuously active during standing (for posture) and in all anti-gravity movements
- Helps to bend the spine backward and twist the body around the spine
- Acts to stabilize the spine during twisting motions

Diaphragm (directly affects how you breath)
- Works with intercostals as the two primary breathing muscles
- Assist in breathing out mainly, as breathing in is largely passive

GLOBAL (PRIME) MOVERS

Rectus abdominis (6-pack)
- Helps you to bend forward and brace your spine by stiffening and pulling towards your centerline
- Helps to tilt the pelvis forward
- Contributes to core stability by working with the transverse abdominis, obliques, and erectors to create a natural weight support belt

External oblique
- Help to rotate the trunk and bend side-to-side
- Helps pull the chest downward (like in a crunch)
- Helps with expelling air

  NOTE: bilateral weakness decreases the ability to bend forward properly, and can lead to hunched posture and an anterior pelvic tilt. This can cause low back pain as well as hip, knee, and ankle issues.

Erector spinae
- Helps to bend the body and head backwards
- Keeps the body from bending forward too fast
- Helps to rotate the head and spine and bend them forward

Short muscles (muscles that have been overworked due to compensation and are too tight) are the primary reason for low back pain. Sometimes these spasms can be debilitating. These muscles are often overworked (too short due to inactivity of the multifidus) and therefore cannot perform the function of stabilizing the spine. This increases the load the spine has to carry, making it easier for the lumbar vertebrae to move excessively or create disc bulges, herniations, or cause the disc to slip out of place.

Quadratus lumborum
- Acts as a cross-road between the forces of neighboring muscles
- Helps to stabilize the diaphragm when breathing in
- Helps to flex the low back side to side safely (for example; when you carry groceries with only one arm the quadratus lumborum helps you to stay upright)
- Connects to hip muscles to stabilize the pelvis

The Quadratus lumborum is considered a postural muscle that helps spare load from the spine. It is also a continuation of the transverse abdominis. When weak, it can contribute to low back pain and/or the hip tilting too much on one side.

CORE HIP MUSCLES

<u>HIP FLEXORS</u>

Gluteus maximus
- Essential for maintaining correct posture
- Helps (with the hamstrings) to stand up from a bent position and to help control your torso as you bend forward.

Glutes can become inactive (and eventually weak if neglected for too long), from being seated for long periods of time. This happens due to the body's energy conservation mechanism. So often, dysfunction of the glute is not necessarily due to weakness, but inactivity. This inactivity leads to an overactive (short and tight) hamstring, which can negatively affect how you walk and can very likely contribute to a fall.

Hamstring
- Plays an important role when walking
- Helps (with the gluteus maximus) to stand up from a bent position and to help control your torso as you bend forward

The hamstring can become very short (or tight) and over-active when seated for long periods of time. This makes it so they cannot properly function and it can have a profound negative effect on how you walk.

<u>HIP ABDUCTORS</u>

Gluteus medius
- Prime mover of outward motion at the hip joint
- Provides opposition while the quadratus lumborum moves to maintain frontal stability of the pelvis

Gluteus minimus
- Works on a deeper level with the gluteus medius to perform the same functions

Tensor Fascia Lata (TFL)
- Works with the gluteus medius and minimus to rotate the hip inward and pull it outward
- It also assists the quadriceps to bend the hip forwards (or bring the knee upwards)

Piriformis
- Assists in sideways rotation of the hip when standing and helps to lift the leg outward when the hip is bent forward

Sartorius
- It helps the hip to bend forward and plays a small role in lifting and rotating the leg outward
- It also plays a small role in bending the leg at the hip when the knee is already bent

Top fibers of gluteus maximus
- These fibers assist lifting the leg outward

All of these muscles provide pelvic stabilization during standing, using stairs, walking, jogging, or running. In fact, they provide nearly three quarters of the pelvic stability in the body!

UPPER QUADRANT – These muscles fire off after the core is activated. They have their own specific functions but secondarily will aid in stability (at the shoulder and shoulder blade) even when performing their primary functions. When a joint near the spine is unstable the core must put forth more energy to those areas to stabilize, leaving the spine less protected.

Trapezius (mobilizer)
- Due to its long fibers that span the back, it is able to assist in nearly all movement where we need postural stabilization assistance
- More specifically, it provides spinal stabilization to keep us standing upright

Supraspinatus, Infraspinatus, and Teres Minor (stabilizers, also three of four muscles of the rotator cuff)
- These muscles help hold the upper part of the upper arm bone (humerus) against the front of the shoulder blade (scapula) to allow postural stabilizers to more effectively stabilize the core and not have to use their energy for shoulder stabilization as the arm moves.

Teres major (mobilizer)
- Sometimes called the "lats little helper" this muscle aids the Latissimus dorsi in extending and internally twisting the arm, as well as drawing it across the body
- It also helps to accelerate the arm (along with the latissimus dorsi) through throwing motions such as when throwing a baseball or chopping motions.

Latissimus dorsi (stabilizer and mobilizer)
- This muscle assists in moving the trunk forward and upward when the arms are overhead and fixed such as when climbing or getting something down from a high shelf

- Additionally, in activities where one would have to use crutches (and the upper arm is fixed in place) this muscle helps to pull the trunk forward relative to the arms to create forward motion.

Stabilizer muscles hold onto bone for postural control and mobilizer muscles primarily move the bones they are attached to.

POSTERIOR OBLIQUE SUBSYSTEM (POS)
Connection between the upper and lower quadrant of the body that runs diagonally from the gluteus maximus (back hip) to the latissimus dorsi (top corner of back)
- Is used anytime you make a movement such as a golf swing, hit a ball with a bat, or perform any outward rotating pulling motion.
- Is used to stabilize the lumbar spine (low back), the sacroiliac joint (where the lower spine and pelvis meet), and the hip.

The posterior oblique subsystem is often underactive (too long), leading to over activity of the AOS

ANTERIOR OBLIQUE SUBSYSTEM (AOS)
Connection between the lower quadrant that runs diagonally from the external oblique (side of the abdomen) and adductors (inner thigh).
- Is used anytime you make a movement such as throwing a ball, pushing against something, a butterfly stroke in swimming.
- Is used primarily in pushing, rotation movements, especially inward movements.

INTRINSIC STABILIZATION SUBSYSTEM (ISS)
Though not recognized as a "true" subsystem, this group of muscles works together in a similar fashion to the other subsystems. They consist of your intrinsic core stabilizers. While this subsystem doesn't significantly contribute to movement, it's imperative that your ISS is strong for optimal movement of any kind and will take work away from the AOS if this subsystem is compromised in any way.

Its main function is to be able to create the proper amount of intra-abdominal pressure to protect the spine when movement occurs or you are trying not to move too much.

This subsystem fires first before any movement from the limbs occurs.

Cueing an abdominal drawing in maneuver has been shown to preferentially recruit the transverse abdominis (TVA) and can be used to create a more effective contraction from the TVA during more functional tasks and specific training.

What is the core used for?
The primary function of the core is to help us breathe properly. Breathing is debatably one of the more important functions of our bodies and the foundation for postural control and control during dynamic movements of any kind. Without proper breathing patterns, your postural stabilizers (pelvic floor, transverse abdominis, internal obliques, diaphragm, and multifidus) cannot optimally activate. Additionally, they cannot activate as precisely in the order in which they are supposed to. They should activate before the global movers (rectus abdominis, external oblique, erector spinae, and quadratus lumborum). When out of sequence, they put load onto

neighboring muscles, tendons, and ligaments that are not designed to handle the kind of work they are being given. It is akin to giving an adolescent a chainsaw and asking them to cut down a tree! It might happen but they'lll be very much worse for wear and it simply isn't a good idea. Consequently, proper breathing mechanics by sequential firing of the postural stabilizers is the precondition to effectively activate the inner core of the spine[5].

Yet another primary function of the core is ultimately to protect the spine, our organs, and keep us upright. It keeps the spine unloaded as forces transfer between the upper and lower body and vice versa. If there isn't optimal firing of the muscles in sequence to create the all-around stiffness around the spine the load can affect it in many negative ways. For example; an inordinate amount of lower back pain is associated with weak postural stabilizer muscles as well as the lower quadrant accessory muscles such as the gluteus maximus. Low back pain can also come from issues at the base of the neck, the multifidus, or the upper quadrant accessory muscles, the latissimus dorsi, or trapezius. Have you ever picked up a heavy box, swung your grandkid around in the air, or even just twisted down to the side to put a dish in the dishwasher? Have you ever done that and felt "something", a twinge, a pull, or maybe more? That sensation of a twinge, pull, or even pain is due most likely to a muscle that was used when it shouldn't have been or it's a weak muscle that cannot stabilize or does not have the stabilization it needs to work effectively. Injuries like this, if severe enough, can put a person out for days to years and in some situations require surgery.

The bottom line is the muscles of the torso (as ALL muscles of the body) have an agonist-antagonist relationship. This means that all muscles have an opposing muscle and without this opposition neither muscle can function properly as they work to speed movement up and slow movement down at the same time to create a balance between the two muscles. This is what allows us to control our movement. In the end, they all must work together as a system to deflect forces around the spine instead of through it. If we fail to keep balance in these muscles it can result in strain being placed on muscles that aren't built for that job or function. Core stabilization comes down to the simple principle of "proximal stiffness to create distal motion (McGill).

CHAPTER 2 – Advantages of Core Exercise

Core exercises are remarkably important for your body and overall health. Your spine, pelvis, and trunk are akin to the chassis of your car. Without that strong platform, it wouldn't last nearly as long or be as safe if you were in an accident. In my experience, seniors with a strong and stable core typically live longer, higher quality lives, have less falls and injuries, and stay independent and mobile for longer. While building a strong core might be daunting, implementing a few fundamental movements and routines can set you on the right path.

The Importance of Core Exercises for Seniors

Hello, fall prevention! If you've already fallen, or feel unstable when walking then core exercises should be top of mind. A strong core means more stability and mobility. Sadly, once a fall occurs, individuals tend to restrict their activity and their strength slowly declines, worsening the problem.

Balance, also known as postural stability, is a generic term that describes the process in which the body's position is maintained in equilibrium. Balance can be stationary, like sitting upright in a chair, or moving, like walking down the hallway. It also incorporates other body systems, including the vestibular, visual, and proprioceptive systems. Each system benefits from specific exercises, but the overall goal is the same. For example, if you're training your upper body at the gym, you don't rep out a few dumbbell curls and call it a day. Many different muscles comprise the upper body, and each muscle needs exercises that appropriately target each one. The bottom line is that to move around safely, there needs to be coordination between all systems in the body.

Even something as simple as standing up straight requires a great amount of strength. Good posture includes the pelvic floor, transverse abdominis, internal obliques, multifidus, and diaphragm that act as scaffolding for the body. The ability of these muscles working together results in mobility, like getting out of bed, hopping into the car, stepping sideways, or stopping the forward motion of your body to stand still. Weakness in any of these areas leads to a breakdown of the system and the foundation that keeps you upright! Sadly, this often prompts a cascade of events that can lead to discomfort, pain, and potentially injury, which will only perpetuate if ignored.

Common signs of poor posture;
-Pain in the following areas – jaw, shoulders, elbow, wrist, hip, knee, ankle, and foot
-Plantar fasciitis
-Migraines

Our weight, or where we hold our weight, can also impact our core strength. Weight control is on all of our minds these days, whether it's weight loss (more so) or weight gain (this happens too!). If our core is strong, our bodies don't have to put as much effort into maintaining balance or preventing a fall (which consumes more energy than you might even be aware of). Instead, that energy can be used to add an extra mile to your walk or going bowling with friends. The result is better mobility and a more fulfilling life.

However, if our core is weak and we hold excess weight in our midsection, we'll likely experience pain, discomfort, and a lack of mobility or flexibility. Keeping your weight in mind is important for posture, but also for our overall health. According to the Mayo Clinic, belly fat is linked to hypertension, sleep apnea, heart disease, and diabetes and increases your chances of certain cancers, stroke, and early death.

Sadly, ailments such as high blood pressure (HBP), stroke, cardiovascular disease (CVD), type 2 diabetes, and other metabolic conditions are all too common in today's world. I can guarantee that nearly everyone has or knows someone with one or more of these diseases. Outside of the physical and mental anguish these diseases can cause, they also take a chunk out of your bank account!

According to the CDC, hypertension and its treatments cost Americans $131 to $198 billion each year9, and this doesn't include the cost of lost productivity! $327 billion was spent on the cost of medical care and lost productivity for those diagnosed with diabetes (CDC). Even more so, those diagnosed with cardiovascular disease cost our healthcare system $216 billion annually and caused $147 billion in lost productivity on the job (CDC)! For nonfatal falls, Medicare paid approximately $28.9 billion, Medicaid $8.7 billion, and private and other payers $12.0 billion. Overall, medical spending for fatal falls was estimated at $754 million (NIH, 2018).

Exercising in general can help you manage, and in some cases reverse, these conditions if you already experience them. If you aren't already exercising, the best time to start is now! As we've already discussed, it's great for mental, physical, social and emotional health!

High blood pressure increases stress on the heart and arteries to an enormous amount and commonly leads to cardiovascular disease (CVD). As high blood pressure chips away at the arteries, fat deposits can get stuck in microscopic tears of the artery wall. A lot of this comes from LDL, or "bad" cholesterol in the bloodstream. This is how plaques build up, and can create a positive feedback loop. Note: In nature, a positive feedback loop occurs when the product of a reaction leads to an increase in that reaction. A narrowed artery, due to plaque buildup, only creates an environment that increases blood pressure, which damages the arteries more, so on and so forth. This can create difficulties in the form of strokes as well. Strokes result from a blood clot inside the brain that obstructs blood and oxygen from circulating, resulting in tissue death, often on one side of the body. Other contributing factors include high blood pressure, CVD, and type 2 diabetes (high blood glucose). All of these conditions share certain attributes that exercising regularly can often reverse. For example, exercising increases the body's ability to uptake glucose (sugars) into the muscles to be utilized and help control LDL cholesterol in the body. With more control of blood sugar and cholesterol, there is less of a risk that excess sugar will cause damage to the artery walls. This keeps blood pressure down and, therefore, your risk for plaque buildup and, consequently, a heart attack or stroke.

Additionally, exercise is brain food. Moving our bodies promotes neurogenesis. Neurogenesis is the development of brain cells and it specifically happens in the hippocampus. The part of the brain that governs memory and learning. Exercise also protects the nervous system from injury and neurodegenerative diseases that can degrade our quality of life or shorten longevity. Exercise also enhances learning and memory functions, increasing brain volume in areas implicated in executive processing.

If you're feeling burnt out lately and don't have a clear cause (work stress, family life or relationships), being out of shape or having a weak core could be the culprit. The weaker our muscles are the less efficient our movements are, resulting in a lot of wasted energy. When the muscular system works optimally, it expends less energy throughout the day, leaving that reserve for other things. Not only do you get to tap those reserves, but through exercise, you will typically receive higher quality of sleep, which lets the body recover from daily tasks better, leaving you with more energy for the next day. If that isn't motivation to start working out, I don't know what is!

We can't talk about muscular health without talking about bone health too! Our muscles move our skeleton around, but without our bones' structural support, our muscles wouldn't have much to move. According to the National Institute on Aging, osteoporosis affects 1 in 5 women over 50 and 1 in 20 men over 50 (NIH, 2022). Osteoporosis causes bones to become weak or brittle, and there are often no signs or symptoms until something goes wrong and you fracture or break a bone, so it's often referred to as a silent disease. Something as mild as a powerful cough or running into the corner of a wall can cause a bone to break or fracture. Even worse, a stress fracture (a crack in the bone due to repetitive pressure. Most commonly occurring in weight-bearing bones like the lower leg and foot, these fractures can rear their ugly heads and cause all sorts of trouble, pain, and discomfort. Not to mention, broken bones lead to a huge disruption in your daily life. Regular weight-bearing exercise as well as impactful exercise (think jumping and landing) can keep bones strong and even reverse some bone loss!

When we think of exercise's positive effects, we typically think more about our physical body. What about our emotions and mental health? Everything we do physically begins in the brain, so mental health plays a direct role in how good our physical health is. Regular exercise increases dopamine (our reward or "feel good" hormone) and endorphins (a calming hormone) production and can decrease cortisol (stress hormone). Exercise can improve self-esteem, your sense of self-accomplishment, and even your coping abilities. It can also distract you from negative thoughts and help promote positivity in general through goal creation and accomplishment.

It would seem there isn't a lot that regular exercise can't do for the body! While not a fix-all, it's most certainly the foundation of the solutions to most physical and mental problems we face.

Benefits of Having a Strong Core

As you can see, there are numerous advantages to exercising in general, and a strong core is the icing on the cake. Let's take a look at some other benefits of exercising.

When you have a strong core, you are using one of the most effective tools in your body to decrease pain or keep pain away overall. This is one benefit that those who have strong and stable core musculatures share. Think about the last time you went to a church gathering, fair, amusement park, or out-of-town shopping center with family or friends. How long were you able to walk around without feeling exhausted, discomfort, or pain? If you could walk around with little to no negative issues, congratulations! You're strong and stable enough to handle the things you do on a daily basis and any extras that come along! However, if your answer was only an hour or so, there is likely room for improvement! Strong core stabilizers, like the *multifidus* and *erector spinae*, make it easier to maintain good posture and support your spine. This means more energy can be used to keep you moving around pain and discomfort free!

If you are strong and stable at the foundation, your body uses existing energy to keep you upright as you stand still and move around. This increases your balance's integrity, diminishing your risk for falls. Typically, this gives you a mental boost of confidence to feel safe and comfortable walking around for more extended periods, too. So, when you are at a busy place, where there is a greater chance you will experience things such as crowds, uneven terrain or stairs, you are able to spend more time at these places with friends, family, or even just on your own!

As you are able to be involved in more and more experiences with less (or no) pain and discomfort, you will become stronger with the movements your body needs to perform more frequently. This means the more muscle memory your body will have to maintain the balance you have acquired by exercising, which can lead to fewer and fewer falls or near falls. This contributes to the positive feedback loop of having a strong core and stabilizing core musculature and all the benefits that comes with it.

Maintaining a social life, friendships, and relationships with family is a cornerstone characteristic of a high quality life. Remaining mobile and independent is one of the best ways to have the flexibility and opportunity to support these types of relationships. Having the physical support you need to keep your body healthy and moving is so important. Your physical and mental well-being increases. Additionally, the amount of help you might need as you age can decrease as you become (and stay) stronger and more able to do day-to-day activities. This increased independence often means more frequent and fun experiences with friends and family.

See how many benefits there can be to having a strong and stable core? It's the beginning of a waterfall of positive benefits. You build and maintain a strong core, which inevitably leads to less pain and discomfort overall. This typically results in better balance and stability, keeping your risk of falling lower than it otherwise would be. This, then leads to you becoming (or remaining) more independent and mobile, which gives you more mental and physical confidence. This becomes self-perpetuating. With a better mental and physical status; you are stronger and suffer less from ailments such as hypertension, CVD, Diabetes, neurodegenerative issues, depression, anxiety, and a myriad of other ailments. Ideally, this means you are more inclined to maintain a strong core (and exercise more). That being said, your ability to exercise is very much dependent on how much core strength you have and how stable it is, which further perpetuates every one of the benefits mentioned above. Remember, you have the power to change your life and get stronger if you choose to. There are innumerable benefits to doing this, and the hope is that this book will help you to achieve many (if not all) of these benefits.

CHAPTER 3 - What Can Happen If You Don't Workout?

A sedentary lifestyle is one of the most common traits among individuals with health problems and can negatively impact many other areas of your life. This can range from sleep and energy to cardiovascular disease, hypertension, type II diabetes, poor mental health, altered gut microbiome, a weakened immune system, and all the way down to our hair, skin and nail health. Immobility is often the start of many of these physical and mental issues. What's even more disheartening is that these ailments characteristically perpetuate a sedentary lifestyle. That waterfall effect will keep going until YOU decide to take control and put a stop to it.

In 2021, hypertension was the primary driving cause of almost 700,000 deaths in the United States! That's a little over 2,000 Boeing 777 airplanes filled with people! Talk about a whole lot of people! We're likely all familiar with the 120/80 blood pressure standard, but nearly half of all adults, or around 120 million, are defined as having a systolic pressure of above 130 mmHg or a diastolic pressure of above 80 mmHg.

Systolic blood pressure, the top number, measures the force the heart exerts on the walls of the arteries each time it beats. Diastolic blood pressure, the bottom number, measures the force the heart exerts on the walls of the arteries in between beats (Mayo Clinic). High blood pressure damages the arteries as the increased pressure of the blood going through the artery creates micro-tears or nicks in the artery walls. Over time, this causes inflammation and plaque buildup, so blood cannot pass through arteries as effectively. This happens because plaque gets caught on those little nicks or micro-tears in the arteries, preventing any artery damage from healing effectively, allowing more inflammation in the body. Over time, these issues can lead to an aneurysm (occurs when part of an artery wall weakens, allowing it to balloon out or widen abnormally) that has the potential to rupture, causing internal bleeding. They can occur anywhere, but the most common areas include the aorta (the main blood vessel carrying blood from the heart to the body), the brain, and behind the knee.

High blood pressure can also lead to an enlarged heart or heart failure if left untreated, not to mention TIA's (transient ischemic attacks or mini-strokes), full-blown stroke, vascular dementia, and mild cognitive impairment. It can even damage major organs like the kidneys due to a lack of oxygen-rich blood reaching the organs. You can develop neuropathy (a term for nerve damage or impairment that can affect any part of the body) in the eyes, hands, and feet. This damage to the blood vessel can become so bad that the nerves around that artery eventually die from lack of oxygen-rich blood. This means the nerves don't work at all, and unfortunately, they don't grow back. This can even lead to issues like sexual or erectile dysfunction. If you think about how important water is to a garden, that is how important blood flow is to our body. If the hose is kinked, even briefly, it can have negative consequences. Over time, that area of the kinked hose weakens and could cut off even more water to your garden. Eventually, the plants don't get enough water and simply die. The biggest difference between our bodies and the plants is that those things affected by lack of blood flow don't necessarily get better or grow back, as in the example with our nerves.

Like the analogy above, coronary artery disease affects the heart more specifically and is exacerbated by hypertension. The major blood vessels that supply the heart (coronary arteries) struggle to send enough blood, oxygen, and nutrients to the heart muscles. Cholesterol deposits (plaques) in the heart's arteries, as well as inflammation, are usually the cause of coronary artery disease. Signs and symptoms only occur when the heart doesn't get enough oxygen-rich blood. If you have coronary artery disease, reduced blood flow to the heart can cause chest pain (angina) and shortness of breath. When a complete blockage of blood flow occurs, that is called a heart attack or myocardial infarction (MI). Coronary artery disease often develops over decades, and symptoms may go unnoticed until a significant blockage causes problems or a heart attack occurs. According to the CDC, coronary heart disease is the most common type of heart disease, killing 375,476 people in 2021. This is why following a heart-healthy lifestyle can help prevent coronary artery disease[14], and why prevention plans almost always include exercise, among other things.

Good and bad cholesterol, though clinical terms, have been a part of common day language for a while now. Most can even tell you the basic difference between good cholesterol or high-density lipoprotein (HDL) and bad cholesterol or low-density lipoprotein (LDL). Both exist in the body naturally and are a combination of protein and fat, and both even have jobs in the body! High-density lipoprotein has a high ratio of protein and very little fat, while low-density lipoprotein has a higher ratio of fat and very little protein. The specific protein and fat combination are needed to move different types of cholesterol around in the body. This is due to the makeup of cholesterol and its attachments, which are not soluble in water (which is what our bloodstream is mostly composed of). We want higher levels of high-density lipoprotein in the body because their main function is to carry cholesterol away from the bloodstream by taking it to the liver for excretion as waste. We want lower levels of low-density lipoprotein overall because if its job is overdone, the end result is plaque buildup. Its primary function in the body is to carry cholesterol into the bloodstream so it can be moved around the body to where it is needed for cell repair by depositing it inside artery walls. However, we only need so much, and when those levels become too high, it can, and does, contribute to plaque buildup. Too much of a good thing can be bad, as this will exacerbate most heart-related issues including coronary artery disease, stroke, and high blood pressure. There is good news that will keep your levels of cholesterol where they ought to be. A review of numerous studies and meta-analyses showed a direct benefit to the increase of high-density lipoprotein cholesterol and a decrease of low-density lipoprotein cholesterol associated with certain types of exercise[15].

When we think about health, we usually think about physical fitness, but cognitive and mental health are huge components of our overall wellness and shouldn't be overlooked. There's currently a vast amount of research focusing on this, especially as baby boomers age into the 65+ category. Cognitive decline is the leading cause of dementia, which has already become a global burden. A sedentary lifestyle is a common precursor to cognitive decline. New studies have even linked glycemic control (blood sugar control) to brain health. The human brain only makes up about 2% of the body's weight but consumes about 20% of the energy the body needs just to survive. Most of this energy is created by utilizing glucose (sugar or carbohydrates) as food. In fact, glucose is the primary energy source for the central nervous system and the brain. In 2018, UCLA researchers found that sedentary behavior is a significant predictor of thinning of the medial temporal lobe (where the hippocampus is located). This is the brain region responsible for the formation of new memories and learning. Medial temporal lobe thinning can be a precursor to cognitive decline and dementia in middle-aged and older adults. Reducing sedentary behavior may be a possible target for strategies designed to improve brain health in people at risk for Alzheimer's disease[16]. A paper published in 2017 in *Alzheimer's & Dementia: Translational Research & Clinical Interventions* journal, found that sedentary nature is linked with poor glycemic control and contributes to overall mortality. While they focus on glycemic control and brain function, the sedentary nature of people appears to be the common denominator[17]. The best way to manage both a sedentary lifestyle, declining cognition, and blood glucose is . . . you guessed it, exercise.

Speaking of blood sugar control, a sedentary lifestyle also contributes to the formation of Type 2 diabetes, according to the American Diabetes Association. Exercise in the short term can drop blood glucose levels for up to 24 hours or more. However, more consistent exercise can positively affect blood sugar control for longer, even lowering your A1C, an average measure of blood sugar over 2-3 months. Specifically, it measures what percentage of hemoglobin proteins (where the iron in your blood is carried) in your blood are coated with sugar. Hemoglobin proteins in red blood cells transport oxygen[18]. The higher your A1C level, the poorer your blood sugar control and your risk of diabetes complications.

Consistent exercise is the best way to manage these complications. Exercise does this by increasing how much sugar the muscle can take from your bloodstream. The more sugar it can take up, the more glucose readily available to your body[19]. Type 2 diabetes is studied extensively, and for good reason. It affects 37.3 million people—that's 11.3% of the US population, and 1 in 5 don't know they have diabetes! 26.4 million adults 65 or older have prediabetes. If you are diagnosed as prediabetic, your blood sugar is higher than it should be but not so high to consider it type 2 diabetes. But don't let that fool you, prediabetes can damage the body nearly as much as the full-blown diagnosis. The hope for prediabetics is they can reverse it through lifestyle changes, namely exercise and healthy food choices. The more control you have over your blood sugar, the less damage will be done to your arteries. We know this means fewer incidences of heart or other major organ issues, not to mention your eye health and retaining the nerves in your hands, fingers, feet, and toes.

One of the greater-known side effects of a sedentary lifestyle is growing physically weaker, or atrophying. When our muscles aren't being used, the body will either make them smaller, resulting in loss of muscle mass, or in some cases get rid of some of the muscle fibers by breaking them down altogether. The purpose for this muscle loss is the body attempting to conserve energy. Does the phrase "use it, or lose it" ring a bell? Because muscle takes a lot of energy to maintain, if the body doesn't have to expend the energy to maintain them, it won't.

In our older years, this is called sarcopenia. Sarcopenia is the age-related progressive loss of muscle mass and strength. The main symptom of the condition is muscle weakness. Sarcopenia is a type of muscle atrophy primarily caused by the natural aging process. Scientists believe being physically inactive and eating an unhealthy diet can contribute to the disease[20]. Muscles are critically important to our overall health and quality of life. They are what keep us mobile and independent, and offer stability to our joints. Unstable joints can lead to many issues, such as arthritis. So, it isn't too irrational to say that arthritis is best managed through a stable joint. This is why strength training is recommended for those who have arthritis. Even if you don't have arthritis, unstable joints can lead to other issues. With unstable joints, you are more likely to fall or become injured, leading to greater complications in the movement you rely on to stay able and independent. Your muscles can become stiffer and less flexible, which causes imbalances and issues all their own. Joint instability will almost always lead to some type of pain and discomfort in the long run. Sadly, we see these as just another part of life, but it doesn't necessarily have to be.

Imagine for a moment that you went out, bought a new bike and rode it regularly for a number of years. Then, for some reason you can't remember, you stopped riding your bike. It just sits outside in the elements, not being ridden or maintained. In a couple of years, you go back to ride it. Except now, the gears are a little wonky, it's rusty and dirty. It's a little harder to pedal as the chain has become stiff, so you have to use a lot more energy to get it to do the same things it did when you first got it. You might be able to ride it again, but it may never ride as it used to. This is akin to what the body goes through when you allow a sedentary lifestyle to take hold. You can get the bike back up to riding shape, but it takes some work and commitment. You have the power to do that. This is best achieved through exercise, and more specifically, core strength and stability. The positive effects of exercise are nearly endless. Exercise is the resolution to many of the issues that ails us, both mentally and physically.

CHAPTER 4 - Safety Precautions & Guidelines Before You Begin

First and foremost, let's begin with stretching. Muscle flexibility and joint mobility are at the center of physical health. Our bodies are constantly searching to strike an equilibrium - even when doing seemingly simple tasks like standing still, lying down, or walking. Your entire musculoskeletal system must be in sync to achieve balance and movement.

Funny enough, while most of us have to work at improving flexibility, a number of people are hypermobile or too flexible. If you fall into this category, be careful, and practice restraint when performing the stretches and exercises mentioned, as laxity in the joints can also lead to injury.

There are numerous types of stretching: static, dynamic, PNF (proprioceptive neuromuscular facilitation), ballistic, active, and passive. We will focus on static and dynamic stretching for our purposes, and the good news is that these are familiar to most folks.

Static stretching occurs when a muscle is lengthened close to its end range, held for a set amount of time (typically 30-90 seconds), and released back to rest. For individuals over 60 years old, it's most effective to hold each stretch for a minimum of 60 seconds[21]. For the perfectionists out there, it's not necessary to push your muscles to complete lengthening. Stretching should never cause pain. Use this as an opportunity to listen to your body. Static stretching before exercise fell out of favor a number of years ago, as it is seen largely as a relaxation activity[22]. While it won't likely cause you a ton of issues, it's best to keep it towards the end of your exercises once your muscles are already warmed up, or perform them on their own.

Dynamic stretching is essentially stretching the muscle through movement. Each exercise will move the muscle through its full range of motion in a slow and controlled manner. More specifically, to get the most out of dynamic stretches, you want them to mimic what you are going to be doing. Not only does it encourage blood flow to the area and warm it up, but it helps create a movement pattern that your brain will recognize so you move better as you head into your activity. It helps excite the muscles more and can increase power and coordination.

Stretching does a lot of good things for the body. It increases circulation to the area you are stretching, increasing the amount of oxygen and nutrients available. Other added benefits of stretching are that it can boost your mood and focus, relieve tension headaches and stress, calm the mind, and even help you sleep better[23]! Additionally, stretching can improve performance, decrease risk of injuries, enable muscles to work more efficiently, and increase your ability to perform activities of daily living independently. A word of caution: stretching should not be considered a warm-up. You should perform foam rolling activities or light cardio for 5-10 minutes, and then you can safely and effectively stretch.

Foam rolling is often seen as something just for athletes, but that couldn't be farther from the truth. Foam rolling, or myofascial release, is self-massage in a nutshell. It is a massage technique that targets the tough membranes that encompass and connect your muscles

21

together, called fascia. If you have ever seen meat with a sheen to some of the tissue, that's the fascia! Anyone who has had a massage will tell you how relaxing and helpful this release of tension can be.

There are numerous benefits to massage, whether done by yourself or with the help of a physical or massage therapist. Massage helps relieve tension and improve circulation, resulting in decreased muscle stiffness and joint inflammation, less pain, improved sleep and recovery, decreased frequency of headaches, improved mood, stress, and energy levels, and helps with things like anxiety and depression (Mayo Clinic Health System, 2022). Self-massage may not be as ideal as someone else helping you out, but you can still reap these benefits and for a lot less money. There are many different types of foam rollers and other tools on the market.

Foam Rollers –
- Smooth or nubby (nubby is good for trigger points overall, mostly up to preference)
- 36" and 18" long (the shorter one is good for traveling, but both work great)
- Soft, medium, and hard density (go with medium or soft if you have very tender skin/muscles)
- Full round, half-round, and almond shapes
- Some vibrate (this may be a nice feature but not necessary)

Stick Massagers –
- Flat surface or multiple independent rollers
- Some allow you to change the configuration of the small independent rollers
- All are great, so much of this is up to preference

Massage Balls –
- Smooth, spiky, nubby (all are good, but nubs and spikes are good for trigger points)
- Tennis balls work great, as do lacrosse and even golf balls (just don't put these directly on your spine)

NOTE: A note on golf balls; they are very hard with no give and are not the first tool you should try when implementing foam rolling, but they can be useful with really tough knots. Take it easy, slow, and steady.

For those who cannot get up and down from the floor, you can still benefit from foam rolling. If you want to use a traditional foam roller, I would recommend a shorter one, as it is easier to use. Place it between you and a wall, leaning into it as you roll, rock, or hold. You can also place it on top of your bed or couch and sit on it like you would on the floor. If you want more pressure, place a book or piece of plywood on the seat of the couch to provide a hard surface for the foam roller to rest on. Though, a stick roller or massage ball may be the easier way to do this. A stick roller is relatively easy to use. You hold it like a rolling pin and use it nearly the same way! With a massage ball, sometimes dropping it into a sock can be helpful when you are trying to massage your back or just to keep a better hold of it.

There are a few rules of thumb when foam rolling. NEVER roll a hurt or bruised muscle, a bone, or a joint. Stick to the muscle belly, which is typically between the joints of the body. Like stretching, it should never hurt, and you should be able to stay relaxed and breathe normally. Roll, rock, or hold for around 30-60 seconds.

Here are a few key components to keep in mind as you stretch:

- *Strive for symmetry:* focus on flexibility equally on both sides of your body. Whatever stretches you perform on one side of your body should be repeated in equal number on the other side of your body.
- *Focus on major muscle groups:* those are the big guys that do the most work, especially those you use a lot (for example, your hips and shoulders)
- *Don't bounce:* bouncing when stretching can often push the muscle well past its normal length and cause injury or damage to the muscle.
- *Remember to breathe:* This does two things. First, you remember to breathe - oxygen is a wonderful thing! Second, slow and deep breathing in through your nose and out through your mouth signals your nervous system to relax and calm down, which can make your stretching more effective[25]
- *Don't aim for pain:* you want to stretch until you feel tension (and maybe a smidge past), but it should NEVER hurt
- *Make your stretches specific:* perform stretches that will mimic what activity you are going to be doing so you can perform that activity better. For example, bending down to pick up groceries or a grandbaby.
- *Keep it up:* Even as little as two to three 10 minute sessions per week can give you great benefit. Unless you keep at it though, you will lose many of those benefits[26]

Another important aspect of stretching to keep in mind if your form and body mechanics. Good form is achieved through stretched, warmed-up muscles and takes a lot of practice. This is the technical part of exercising or activity. Bad form can potentially cause serious injury, especially to the spine, and a strong core with good stability won't always protect you. Furthermore, bad form tends to work the wrong muscles or work them in a way they aren't supposed to move. This can be frustrating if you work towards a specific goal with a certain group of muscles, as it creates a false sense of progress. This false sense of achievement comes, typically, when you perform an exercise through only part of its full range of motion or if you are posed in a way that lets you perform the move more easily than with proper form[27]. Bad form mostly means the execution of your movement is unsafe, inefficient, or both. Bad form doesn't guarantee an injury, nor does good form assure safety. However, good form puts the odds in your favor. Optimal form can vary from person to person as we are all built (or put back together in some cases) differently. However, there are some basics you can stick to to achieve proper or good form[28].

Focus on the work your muscles will be doing, and how you'll be moving. If you are distracted thinking about your lack of sleep from last night, tasks you have to get done later in the day, or bills you have to pay, then your focus will be diminished. This creates a dissociation and prevents that mind-muscle connection from occurring. The result can be bad form, poor movement execution, and in some cases injury.

Make your muscles do all the work. Momentum or gravity should never carry your movement unless it's part of the movement itself. If you can't control your own body weight, you shouldn't be adding extra weight in the form of dumbbells to your exercises. Get used to moving your body so that if you lose balance or something goes awry you're able to correct it before a fall results. Always be aware of your posture and remember that core strength and stability are the foundation for good form.

Remember to breathe. Knowing when and how to breathe is fundamental for good form for several reasons. First, taking a big inhale before beginning a movement creates internal pressure that helps stabilize your core. Hold this breath until the middle of the movement, and focus on slowly exhaling on the way out of the movement. Also, listen to your body. More on this later. Proper form doesn't just apply to an activity or exercise either. It's a necessity and a huge benefit in our day-to-day lives. Remember, it begins with a strong foundation, namely your core.

Increase your repetitions gradually. Our body builds muscle when it has been challenged. The soreness we might feel the day after a difficult workout is actually due to microtears in the muscle tissue that we created on purpose! It sounds a little daffy, but it is what it is. The body senses these microtears, and the systems responsible for repairing this damage spring into action. Soreness is something that nearly everyone has felt at one time or another, some worse than others. I'm sure we can all remember a younger time when we physically pushed ourselves too hard and walking or even holding a cup of coffee the next day was challenging. That's taking things a little too far, and that's not our goal here. The body repairs the microtears we create but makes sure to build them back a little bit better. This is how muscle strength, power, endurance, and size are gained. Only with sufficient rest and nutrition will this happen effectively.

There are several ways to challenge the body, and increasing repetitions is one of them. When increasing a challenge to the body, a good rule of thumb is to go slow and build small. Baby steps are the name of this proverbial game. When you take the time and care to build your challenge up slowly, your body will have less to repair all at once, and you will be able to perform your exercise routine more frequently. If you go too big too fast, you may need to take days or even weeks to rest and recover, and this can seriously set you back. Think like the tortoise, not the hare.

Listen to your body. I know, I know, this sounds like fitness gibberish, but hear me out. Listening to your body is knowing the difference between soreness and pain and understanding how far to push your body. It's knowing when your head isn't in the game and perhaps you need a rest day or a day of light activity[29]. One adage that needs to be retired is, "no pain, no gain". If something hurts, then you need to stop or try something else. Physical activity and exercise should never be painful. It can cause discomfort and, perhaps, toe the line of pain. However, don't mix up the uncomfortable nature of physical activity and pain. Be especially aware if you have neuropathy, as that limits the frequency of signals that go to your brain telling you something is hurt or injured. If your neuropathy is bad enough, your body might not be able to relay these messages at all, so be sure to check those areas of your body often during activity. Furthermore, if you have a high pain tolerance, also tread carefully. A high pain tolerance may seem neat, but it can certainly put a damper on things if you push too far and don't take notice.

Be consistent. Consistency, over nearly every other modality, is one thing those most successful with exercise have in common. It is arguably one of the most important aspects of fitness. When you are consistent with your movement, you gain a ton of knowledge about how you move and feel. These data points will allow you to know your body better through and through. A fascinating side effect of consistency in exercise is that many people begin to know their bodies so well they can predict when they have an illness coming on, such as a cold or the flu. It also makes it easier for you to communicate with any health professionals you see, which means they can determine a better avenue of care for you if there is something wrong. This brain-body connection is incredibly powerful as it's a big part of how to stay mentally able, alert, and ward off diseases such as Alzheimer's and dementia. This aids greatly in neuroplasticity, which is the ability of the brain to form and restructure connections in your nervous system, especially in response to learning or experience or following injury. If you remain consistent, you will see progress.

Now, let's talk about good, high-quality sleep. Recuperation is critical to our way of life, and it has a direct effect on the quality of life we have. Whether you have exercised really hard or just performed your normal day-to-day activities, you need to rest, and recover. I would surmise that rest is almost more important than nearly anything we do for our bodies. Muscle growth (or maintenance) can only be achieved through the body being challenged and then helping it to recover through proper nutrition and high-quality rest. Without this recovery, you can almost look at it as time and energy wasted that you spent in pursuit of bettering yourself.

High-quality rest can be difficult to achieve in today's society, especially in the United States. The world around us moves alarmingly fast, our lives and jobs are stressful, and it's sometimes seen as a weakness to slow down and give our body the rest it deserves. According to Johns Hopkins Medicine, many things can disrupt sleep and, therefore, recovery. Long or late naps, too much caffeine, lack of exercise, too much screen time before bed, certain health conditions, frequent nighttime urges to use the bathroom or incontinence, and certain medications, including those used to treat depression, high blood pressure, heart disease, and many others. The natural sleep changes that occur with age are a little more out of our control, but they can be worked with. For example, people tend to fall asleep later and wake up earlier, spend more time in a lighter sleep cycle, and wake up more frequently at night. This is primarily due to low levels of melatonin and certain growth hormones the body produces.

Poor sleep is linked to a number of health problems commonly experienced by older adults as well, like falls, depression, and dementia. It adds to the difficulty of managing chronic diseases such as diabetes, heart disease, and chronic pain[30]. While there are several things you can't do anything about, there are a fair number of things you can do something about. Regular exercise is one of those solutions that will positively affect nearly everything that may be keeping you from receiving better, high-quality sleep.

Prepare yourself and brace! Bracing is another fitness term that may sound like gobbledygook. However, when performed properly, bracing is the single best way to engage the entirety of the core and to create the stiffness needed to protect the spine. It is the key component to begin ANY exercise or movement that will be challenging. When you learn to brace properly, the extra fun part is that it turns any move into a core exercise! Learning how to brace can be complicated for some and easier for others. When you brace your core, you are engaging your transverse abdominis, a deep core muscle that acts like a belt around the spine in your lower back and helps protect it from pressure and too much load. This muscle is meant to be active (and pretty much is), whether we are lifting something heavy off the floor, getting out of bed, standing around, or exercising.

<u>Bracing – Technique #1</u>
1. Place your hands on each side of your abdomen
2. Take a deep breath in, focusing on expanding your abdominal area
3. As you inhale, you'll feel the muscles on each side of your core starting to expand
4. As you exhale, maintain the engagement of those core muscles. Keep them activated
5. After exhaling, relax your core muscles momentarily. Then, inhale again and repeat the process

This technique, known as deep breathing with core bracing, is highly effective in engaging your core muscles. It helps establish a strong mind-muscle connection, allowing you to feel the engagement using your hands.

Bracing – Technique #2
1. Imagine someone playfully coming to punch you in the belly
2. Automatic bracing: In response to this, your reflexes naturally kick in, causing your core to brace automatically
3. Think of it as if a child is playfully aiming a punch at your abdomen. This imagery helps you instinctively tighten your core muscles
4. Muscle activation through visualization: Visualize this scenario quickly when you need to engage your core. You can also place your hands on each side to feel the expansion

As you become more mindful of these muscles, you'll find engaging and feeling them easier each day[31].

Go beyond the abs. While the core stabilizers and other core musculature are important to obtain high-quality movement, our core isn't much without the other muscles of the body! Those muscles move us around and let us do what we need for survival and to have a good time! A routine that encompasses the whole body is paramount to physical and mental health. A full body routine will make everything you do a little easier and keep you from declining as quickly as you age. Just like the relationship between the core stabilizers that must engage first before the global movers (glutes, hamstrings, hip flexors, trapezius, latissimus dorsi, etc.), your core must be strong along with all of your other muscular systems for you to remain sturdy, mobile, healthy, and independent.

Take it easy and start slowly. Just like increasing repetitions gradually, you want to start things off with a slow roll and add to the challenge only when you've mastered the previous movements. First and foremost, you want to work your core stabilizer muscles (your foundation). You don't build a house from the roof down, do you? Then, you can incorporate your global movers and, eventually, your whole body. Taking things one day, one week, one month at a time is the best way to see results. Small changes typically have the most staying power. When presented with a big goal, we often want to pounce on the opportunity to make the change, but this can easily become overwhelming and even detrimental to our progress.

It isn't bad to have a big goal, in fact, it's very helpful. However, where the magic happens are the small habits and changes we adopt[32]. If your goal is to exercise 5 days per week and you begin with that as your only goal, there is a better chance than not that you'll workout less, if not at all. This can be defeating and frustrating, and not the most productive way to get back into working out. However, if you start with one or two days per week and add an extra day every two weeks, eventually, this activity will become part of your daily routine. This is the difference between a choice and a habit. The idea is that your goal becomes a habit, and you do this by creating a new normal each time you tick off a small step toward your bigger goal.

Other considerations. Exercise and activity should be challenging, but you aren't going to throw it into high gear to begin with. An RPE or rate of perceived exertion is a good way to gauge your exertion level. The RPE scale measures the intensity of your exercise or activity and ranges from 0 – 10 (or 0-20 in some cases). The numbers relate to phrases that rate how easy or difficult you find an activity. For example, 0 (nothing at all) would be how you feel when sitting in a chair; 10 (very, very heavy) is how you feel at the end of an exercise that takes all of your energy or after a very challenging activity. This is a subjective scale that anyone can use to gauge their level of exertion. As you begin, you want to aim for the 3-4 range and work up to the 6-9 range, depending on your overall goal and any physical limitations.

Other factors to consider are hydration and nutrition. Water is vitally important to our body functions, as is the food we consume. The National Council on Aging recommends about 1/3 of your body weight in ounces of water each day as a minimum. For example; if you weigh 150lbs, you want to drink about 50 ounces of water daily. This is a guideline; you may find you need more or less. It's good to talk to your doctor about how much water you should be drinking. Additionally, getting enough carbohydrates, fats, protein, vitamins, and minerals is something you should also pay attention to. Protein is especially important. The current RDA (recommended dietary allowance) is 0.8g of protein per kilogram of body weight per day. So, for that same 150lb person, they would want to aim for roughly 55g of protein per day.

Hint: To do this calculation on your own, take your weight in pounds and divide it by 2.2. This will give you your current weight in kilograms. Then multiply that number by 0.8 to get how much protein you should aim to consume each day.

Older adults typically eat too little protein, which is integral to warding off muscle loss and maintenance or gain. 38% of adult men and 41% of adult women have dietary intakes below the recommended amounts[33]. It's no wonder those in the fitness industry recommend closer to 1.2-2g of protein per kilogram of body weight per day. Additionally, eating enough carbohydrates (mostly whole grains), fats (mostly plant-derived sources), plenty of fiber, lots of produce, less processed foods, and foods with added sugars will keep your body on the right track!

The bottom line is that you must prepare yourself properly to avoid injury and make beneficial progress towards a stronger core and overall stronger version of yourself!

CHAPTER 5 – Signs & Symptoms of a Weak Core

Signs and symptoms, while unique to each individual, are experienced by every single one of us. They manifest as a result of change in our body or mind and can tell a story, especially when related to pain or discomfort. It is very important to your overall health to pay attention to signs and symptom as they occur. It can be fairly easy to dismiss them as a fluke or happenstance; however, they shouldn't be so willingly ignored. The story your body's signs and symptoms tell you lets you know if something is wrong and where the issue is or stems from. It can be part of the solution as well. Pay attention to your body's signs and symptoms so you can be proactive about your health and take control of your quality of life. There are many signs and symptoms of a weak core, and they are not to be ignored. One perk as it pertains to these signs and symptoms of a weak core . . . most of them have very, very similar solutions, so you can knock many of them out at the same time. Below are some of the most commonly experienced signs and symptoms related to weak core musculature.

You have low back pain

Roughly 3 million people per year are diagnosed with some type of back pain. One upside regarding treatment is that those who experience this back pain can often treat it themselves. Perhaps fortunately, this type of pain is often unrelated to an underlying disease and is more associated with sitting or lying down for prolonged periods of time, having an overall sedentary lifestyle, poor posture, sleeping in an odd position, wearing poorly fitted shoes, overuse, too much movement between the vertebrae, muscles that are too tight or too loose. The list can go on and on. All of which, by the way, can be solved with a strong core.

Symptoms of low back pain can range from a mild, dull ache to a more severe stabbing, shooting, or seizing pain. Stiffness and tightness are common symptoms and can make standing up or sitting difficult. If left uncorrected, this can lead to postural issues affecting walking. For example, you might walk stooped over with a hunch in your upper back. This hunch can actually result in our lower back flattening out, and together, these misalignments can do a number to your spine.

Muscle spasms are another commonly experienced symptom and can occur after training or overusing your back muscles. These spasms can be disruptive, impairing sleep and making it difficult to complete daily tasks[35].

Hamstring issues are common contributors to low back pain as well. If the hamstrings are short and overactive (the most common issue), they pull the pelvis into a posterior tilt. This again flattens out the lower back and over-stretches muscles, including the erector spinae, making them weaker over time. This torsion can also throw off the alignment of your spine, increasing the amount of pressure on each vertebrae involved and making them less effective at absorbing impact during simple things like walking or sitting down. Additionally, a sedentary lifestyle at home and work directly contribute to a lack of innervation to the butt (gluteus maximus), placing excessive pressure on the hamstrings and forcing them to be overactive.

<u>*You lack power and stability during everyday activities.*</u>
The core musculature provides power and stability and is the foundation for any and all movement. In other words…it's pretty important. Simple movements like bed sitting can become quite challenging if you lack core strength. All this extra effort for normally easy tasks will require much more energy, meaning you'll likely feel you have less energy to do things you enjoy. This is largely because the body will prioritize energy to the core to keep the spine as safe as possible, and a strong core makes a significant difference in the quality of your movement.

A few small studies have shown how significantly core strength affects our daily movements. For example, a 2020 study found that individuals with stronger trained cores rotated their pelvis 29% less than those with weaker core muscles, meaning they were better able to control pelvic movement when performing single-leg activities like walking where one foot is in constant contact with the ground[36]. A more stable pelvis translates to a more stable spine.

<u>*There is discomfort when lying on your back.*</u>
Pain or discomfort when lying on your back is a big indicator that your core is weaker than it should be. More specifically, it can mean you have strained or sprained the muscles in your back. The postural muscles (erectors, multifidus, transverse abdominis and more) may be too loose (weak), and/or your front abdominals or hip flexors are too tight (weak) and overworked. Over time, this weakened musculature could result in one or more slipped or bulging discs due to excess movement or instability within the spine itself. You can also develop a pinched nerve from your vertebrae moving how they normally shouldn't. With time, this movement of the spine could even lead to arthritis.

In addition to keeping us upright and protecting the spine, our core muscles are designed to maintain a certain amount of curvature in three different areas of the spine. From the side, our spine has a natural "S" curve to it. This specific curvature allows for an even distribution of weight through our spine and gives it maximum flexibility and movement to do what our bodies need to do while remaining safe and supported[37].

<u>*You have excessive inward or outward curvature of the lower back.*</u>
As mentioned previously, our spine has a natural curvature that allows us optimal movement and stability. The three specific areas are:

Lordotic curve: This is indicated by a front-facing "C" shape and is seen in our upper (cervical) and lower (lumbar) spine.

Kyphotic curve: This is indicated by a backward facing "C" shape and is seen in our mid (thoracic) spine.

Typically, the low back tries to curve too far inward more often than outward, though this can also happen. When the low back curves too far inward, it is commonly called excessive lordosis, or swayback. Physically, this might make someone's buttocks appear more pronounced in the back and their bellies more prominent from the front. Fun fact, you can typically tell if someone suffers from excessive lordosis by looking at their belt. If it looks bent forward, that's often a sign that their posture is affected, and their hips and pelvis are pushing forward more than usual, taking the belt with it. This leads to extreme pressure on the spine over time, making everyday activities challenging, disrupting sleep and other functions. Other things can lead to excessive lordosis as well, such as osteoporosis.

The opposite of this condition is excessive kyphosis. This condition will make the lower back flatten too much. This is less typical than excessive lordosis. You will notice this in people who look like they have little to no curvature of the lower back, or their head or upper body bends forward more so than it naturally would. With excessive kyphosis, there may be pain with activity or with long periods of sitting or standing. Severe kyphosis can even impact lung capacity if the thoracic cavity is crunched forward enough, restricting airflow and lung expansion[38].

You have difficulty when standing from a squat or seated position.

We stand up or squat numerous times throughout the day, whether out of a chair, getting out of bed, or after using the bathroom. We need to squat down and get up when picking something up off of the floor, looking in a cabinet, or getting in and out of a car. Squatting is arguably the most functional activity of our lives. A weak core leads to instability in nearly all we do but can be seen or felt the most when we try to squat, as our bigger muscle groups and joints are weak or unstable. Without a strong core, we tend to squat less and less. Eventually, this motion becomes unfamiliar to our bodies, making it even more challenging and/or painful to perform.

Remember, our bodies will not maintain muscle it doesn't use on a regular basis. Once this muscle loss occurs, it can be tough to get it back. Not only that, the less we are able to squat properly, the more issues arise around other areas of the body. For example, this leads to poor alignment of the thigh bone (femur) as it glides forward over the shin bone (tibia) when the knee bends. Squatting incorrectly can eventually become painful and even lead to damage of the soft tissue around the knee, including the meniscus or collateral ligaments. Wearing over time can lead to early-onset arthritis. It can also lead to poor tracking of the knee cap (patella), which can cause the knee to fold inward (genu valgum; more common) or outward (genu varum; less common). You see the knee folding inwards in many people, especially older adults. This can increase the risk of falls because when the knee folds inward, it causes the feet to cross one another when walking. It can also lead to uneven weight distribution or muscle imbalances. On top of that, we tend to brace in anticipation of pain or discomfort we know will occur as we squat, and this uses a TON of extra energy throughout the days, weeks, and months, leading to fatigue and other issues all on its own[39]. Needless to say, our core muscles and their impairments have wide-reaching impacts on our whole body. A pain or discomfort we may have learned to live with or accept could be fixed by implementing some of the exercises in this book.

Take time to think critically about any ailments you might be experiencing and how they could relate to your core.

You feel off balance and unstable.

While the reality of this might be tough to wrap your head around, if you're feeling unstable or off balance, it's time to get some help. Whether the issue is a weakened core or something else, you should speak with your doctor for your safety.

Core strength preserves your spine's stability, which translates to stability elsewhere in the body. Our body constantly seeks equilibrium in everything we do, and maintaining core strength is the biggest help we can give our body in this process. If you feel unstable or off balance, you are less likely to move as much or in certain ways that would let you live your best life and allow your body to work optimally. In a broader sense, you are less likely to head to unfamiliar places or be able to be out and about on your own, with friends, or with family. You are less likely to maintain activities that will get you and keep you balanced and stable. This lack of confidence in your movement will lead to less and less movement over time or a more sedentary lifestyle. A sedentary lifestyle has magnanimous implications (refer to Chapter 3) that we see so often they are no longer rare or seen as serious. You may feel more fatigued or weaker as your body has to expend more energy to stay upright and stable. You may have muscle pain, spasms, or stiffness because your body is using muscles it shouldn't be to keep you upright or move you around. In a nutshell, if you are unstable and off balance, it leads to many issues with your muscles and skeleton. This leads to even more inactivity, which trends towards reduced function of other systems in your body such as your heart, lungs, and endocrine (hormones), which, in turn, can lead to total body deconditioning[40]. This type of deconditioning is characteristically very, very difficult to come back from, if at all.

You have pain or discomfort in the pelvis.

We discussed how low back pain can be indicative of a weak core a few paragraphs back, but low abdomen pain or pain in the front of the pelvis can occur as well. Typically, this will have to do with your pelvic floor weakening and being underutilized. The pelvic floor forms the base of your core musculature and creates a "bowl" or "sling" of muscles and other soft tissue whose main function is to maintain the continence of urine and feces, and allows voiding, defecation, sexual activity, and childbirth[41]. All of which are pretty important! Symptoms of pelvic floor weakness or dysfunction include urinary issues, such as the urge to urinate or painful urination, constipation or bowel strains, lower back pain, pain in the pelvic region, genitals, or rectum, discomfort during sexual intercourse for women, pressure in the pelvic region or rectum, or muscle spasms in the pelvis[42].

There are many ways to strengthen the pelvic floor muscles and regular core exercises and bracing properly are great tools to do this. A few studies show that increasing strength in the pelvic floor muscles alleviates many of the aforementioned symptoms and can help correct common issues such as incontinence. For example, in 2022, a study found that core exercises in addition to pelvic floor exercises decreased urinary incontinence and leakage by 72% over a 12-week period[43]. That's a huge success!

You have difficulty walking upright.

This is probably one of the most recognizable and universal signs of a weak core. Yes, there can be other reasons why someone cannot walk upright, however, those reasons are usually exceptions. If you, or anyone you see, walks around looking like the letter "C" from the hips to the head, that is a big indicator they have poor core stability and, therefore, bad posture.

If you sway excessively when you walk, you may have a weak core. This swaying can be troublesome as it makes it tougher to carry things, especially one-sided, like a bag of groceries, and can increase your risk of falling down. Everyday tasks can become more challenging as your body uses more energy to keep you upright and stable than it otherwise would. It also happens to be a telltale sign of aging. Individuals with bad posture when walking (or sitting) are not only perceived as older, it actually amplifies the aging process. There is a reason the stereotype exists. Exercising to maintain a strong core and keeping yourself upright as you move around will help keep you feeling and looking younger!

31

CHAPTER 6 – Basic Steps to Developing Your Core

The beginning steps to developing a strong core are not incredibly difficult, though they are most likely foreign to many. The basics often get lost in the shuffle of the "big event", and there's a reason for this. They aren't fancy or exciting; they are often boring and, in the end, no one can tell you've done them, so we feel like we have nothing to show for it. However, they tend to be the most important actions. You wouldn't build your house on a foundation of gravel or sand, so why would you build your body's strength and stability that way? While houses can be torn down and rebuilt, our bodies are with us for life, and we only have one. Let's put preparation and the basic steps at the forefront of our minds as we progress towards a strong foundation.

Prepare your mind. All movement begins in the brain, so it only makes sense we would want to start here and hold space for what we're about to learn. These movements will help our bodies function and move more effectively and with greater power and direction. This is akin to a French culinary expression often used in kitchens called mise én place, meaning "to put in place" or "gather". It refers to the setup and organization of ingredients and tools required before cooking and is an efficient way to prepare food or meals with minimal snafus. Think about doing this within your mind before starting any activity. Do you have everything you'll need to complete this task successfully? If you think through the exercise before doing it, you'll likely have better form and could see improvement sooner, not to mention decrease your risk of injury and error.

Let's begin with the following:
1. *Define your Motivation* - Motivation will come and go, but establishing your WHY will give you the discipline to follow-through with promises you've made to yourself. Why do you want to do this? How does strengthening your core help you? This gives you 100% accountability to YOURSELF. You are in charge of your decisions, successes and inevitable challenges.
2. *Visualize Success* - Humans are unique when it comes to higher thinking and processing power. If you imagine the path that leads you to achieving your goals, they become more and more real and seen as more attainable. This can very much become self-prophesizing, or even a new buzz-word called "manifesting".
3. *Empty your mind* - Pay attention to your breath and allow it to help clear your mind to focus on the task at hand[44]. We're all busy - whether your spouse is yelling for the remote, kids or grandkids need help with homework, the dog needs to be fed, or you have a work deadline or errands to run. While you're working on these core exercises, let everything go. Focus on yourself for a change. All those problems will likely still be there and remain unchanged if you come back to them in 30 minutes. I've been working on this myself. You need to take care of YOU before you can take care of anyone else. Selflessness has been rewarded and admired for so long, but let's change the narrative. You're important. PERIOD. Filling up your own cup will allow you to better fill the cups of those you love. Give yourself time and grace for at least a little moment each day.

Here are some practices to help you stay in the moment while exercising:

5 Elements of Mindful Exercise
- <u>Intention</u>: Physical activity begins well before you actually move. It's a good idea to understand the function of your exercises, have confidence in the performance of your exercises, and understand your goal and your why. Practicing intention will increase the benefit you receive and maximize the time spent doing the activity.
- <u>Breathing</u>: Breathing while visualizing the exercise in your head is a fantastic way to "practice" before you actually perform the movement. Ideally, you breathe in at the beginning of the exercise, steadily let a little breath out during the most strenuous phase, and inhale again at the top of the movement. However, with lighter or less strenuous exercises, focus more on simply breathing and not on when you are inhaling and exhaling.
  For example, in a squat, you'll fully inhale at the top before beginning your descent. Brace your core. Let a little air out as you descend, and blow the rest of the air out as you rise back up, thinking about pushing off the floor. Once you reach the top, you'll fully inhale again and reset for the next repetition.
- <u>Timing</u>: Each exercise has its own natural tempo. Not only that, focus on slow and controlled movement to ensure the correct muscles are being activated. This may actually allow you to see results sooner and also prevent injury.
- <u>Form</u>: Remember, while bad form doesn't guarantee injury, neither does good form guarantee safety. However, with good form, the ball is in your court and will lend itself to a safer exercise experience. Once again, it gives you more benefit from that exercise.
- <u>Recovery</u>: Arguably one of the most important factions of exercise. Not only after your routine but between sets and repetitions as well. This is why remaining present in the moment is so important. Your muscles recover a little bit each time you rest between repetitions or sets. The more in tune you are to this the better your muscles can "recharge" during and after your routine. Not only that, recovery is essential to remaining injury-free[45].

<u>SPINAL MOTION</u>

Having spinal awareness means that, proprioceptively, you have an understanding of and can feel how your spine is moving. Some people can feel this by individual vertebrae, while others have to work on it. For example, if you have any experience deadlifting, you know how important it is to maintain a straight back. If there's any bend, you risk injuring yourself. But it takes practice, as it's not very natural to keep your spine straight at all times.

Additionally, you want to be aware of how your shoulders and pelvis work with the spine to make quality movement possible. The area of our upper body where our shoulders lie is called the shoulder girdle, while our pelvis and hips make up the pelvic girdle. They attach our arms and legs to our trunk via ball and socket joints. This kind of attachment allows for the largest range of motion, but can also be very unstable. Not only that, but tension, pain, or injury in any of these areas can be felt or transferred to other areas of the body due to how interconnected everything is. Imagine you over work your shoulder, and months down the line, even though it has "healed" you now get an ache in the opposite side of your low back or hip. It may not seem like much, but it can make walking or other activities you do throughout the day more difficult or even painful[46]. Additionally, all movement our arms and legs make begins in the spine!

Having a high awareness of the spine and how to control its movement will lead to greater control over time and, thus, greater control over your limbs all around. This ideology is a cornerstone for those in rehab from spinal damage, whether from trauma or congenital issues.

It's used to teach individuals what it feels like when the spine moves properly when lying down, standing, sitting, or moving.

ACTIVITY: Build Awareness of Spinal Motion

While standing for this activity is ideal, you may perform this movement seated. The goal is to bring awareness to your vertebrae and how they feel as they bend, flex, stretch, and activate. If you feel comfortable doing so, close your eyes as this will limit distractions and allow you focus on each movement more. If you close your eyes, make sure you can hold on to something to keep your balance.
1) Stand or sit up tall
2) Beginning with your head, very slowly start to bend forward, imagining moving each vertebra, one at a time.
    a) I recommend counting your vertebra as you go down and back up; you have 7 cervical vertebrae, 12 thoracic vertebrae, and 5 lumbar vertebrae (24 in all)
3) Keep bending forward, one vertebra at a time, and think about how it feels. Only go as far as you can without pain or discomfort. If you can fully bend over without limitation, this movement is similar to bending over to pick something up off the floor.
4) Once you are at your end range, hang out for a few seconds and breathe in and out a few times
5) Once you are ready, reverse the motion slowly, beginning at the base of your spine. Roll yourself up one vertebra at a time, thinking about how it feels. Does it feel different going in the opposite direction?
    a) You want to go slowly for two reasons. One is to remain aware of your spine, and moving slowly draws your attention to this. Also, going slowly limits the amount of blood pressure change you will experience, limiting the potential for dizziness or light-headedness as you rise
6) Once you are upright, take a moment to do a head to toe check and see how you feel overall[47]

PELVIC MOTION

There are two different types of pelvic motion. The pelvis can move as a unit and has intra-pelvic movement or movement within the pelvis. Pelvic movement as a unit lets us tilt our pelvis forwards and backwards, side to side, and lets it rotate left and right (or all around). Imagine a dashboard Hula doll and how the lower portion of the doll moves when disturbed. While our pelvis doesn't move with quite the same amount of pizzazz, it's a good illustration of the directions our pelvis can move because of the spine. The pelvis works hand-in-hand with the spine. This is because the base of the sacrum (fused vertebrae that includes your tailbone) is where the spine sits and the sacrum is attached directly to the pelvis. Therefore, if the posture of the pelvis changes, so does the position of the sacrum and the spine[48]. Pelvic posture is directly related to spinal posture. Ultimately, we want to keep our Hula doll from going crazy!

ACTIVITY: Build Awareness of Pelvic Motion

Control of the pelvis also means control of the low back or lumbar spine.

Forwards and Backwards

1. Sit on a stability ball or quarter-folded bath towel
2. Begin by sitting up nice and tall, focusing on lengthening through the spine. Since you're sitting on an unstable surface, take a moment to feel the motion beneath you.
3. With your hands on your hips, slowly stick your tailbone out behind you and notice how your low back feels (your erectors are pulling backwards and up on your pelvis and your hip flexors are stretching).
4. Slowly reverse this motion and tuck your tailbone underneath you. Again, notice how your low back feels (your abs are pulling forward and up on your pelvis and your glutes are stretching)

Side to Side

During this movement, your hip abductors (gluteus medius and gluteus minimus) are pulling one side of your hip up and the quadratus lumborum is stretching.

1) Stand up tall and hold on to something with your right hand, place your left hand on your left hip
2) Put all of your weight into your right leg and without bending your knee, hike your hip up to get your foot off of the ground, pay attention to how this feels in your back
3) Repeat on the other leg.

   Modified:
   a) If seated, slide to the left side edge of your chair and let your left cheek hang off the edge. Be sure to hold on to something.
   b) Let the left hip drop towards the floor and raise it back up again, pay attention to how this feels in your back
   c) Repeat on the other side

SHOULDER MOTION

Much like the pelvis, our shoulder girdle allows us to utilize our arms and upper body to reach and tilt in all different directions. The shoulder girdle functions as the anchor that attaches the upper limbs to the cervical spine (upper back). Additionally, the shoulder girdle allows for a large range of motion, mainly in the highly mobile scapulothoracic joint (shoulder blades and where they attach to the spine). The shoulders are attached to the spine via the clavicle (collar bone) and scapula (shoulder blades). The scapula is directly attached to the spine via the trapezius muscle, and the upper arm and upper hip are connected by the latissimus dorsi muscle[49].

There are two ways you can build awareness in the shoulders, and both are worth a try.

Variation #1

1) Stand with your back against a wall so your shoulders and butt are touching it
   a) You can also sit in a high back chair, just make sure you are flush against its back
2) Slowly, raise your arms out in front of you and up overhead as far as you can without pain or discomfort
   a) Note: You should feel your mid/upper back come away from the wall. Pay attention to what this feels like.

Variation #2

1) Stand with your back against a wall so your shoulders and butt are touching it

a) You can also sit in a high back chair, just make sure you are flush against its back
2) Beginning with your head, slowly begin to look downward by tilting your head forward and let your shoulders come off of the wall or chair back, pay attention to what this feels like
3) Reset against the wall or in the chair and now slowly press your shoulders into the wall or chair back
   a) Note: You will feel your upper back come away from the wall. Pay attention to how that feels.

PELVIC FLOOR MUSCLE MOTION

Our pelvic floor serves many different important purposes. Remember, our pelvic floor helps us to remain continent, and plays a huge role in optimal sexual function. It supports the lower back, pelvis, and hips as a part of the core and serves as a support system for organs such as the bladder, uterus, and rectum. It also facilitates the circulation of blood and lymph from this area with the rest of the body. When all is said and done, I'd say our pelvic floor deserves the opportunity to stay strong and able.

ACTIVITY: Awareness of the Pelvic Floor

There are two different pelvic floor awareness exercises. Each targets a slightly different area of the pelvic floor so make sure to try them both.

Anterior Pelvic Floor Activation
1. Stand or sit up tall
2. Close your eyes, if you are standing hold on to something so you do not lose your balance
3. Imagine you are urinating (without actually doing the deed), and focus on slowly contracting your pelvic floor to "stop" the flow of urine.
4. Release the contraction slowly imagining the pelvic floor dropping towards the ground or gently bulging as if you are actively relaxing it
Note: You can also think of your vulva or scrotum dropping down towards your feet

Posterior Pelvic Floor Activation
1. Stand or sit up tall
2. Close your eyes, if you are standing hold on to something so you do not lose your balance
3. Imagine you have to pass gas. Slowly contract your pelvic floor muscles to "stop" from passing gas.
4. Release the contraction slowly, imagining the pelvic floor dropping towards the ground or gently bulging as if you are actively relaxing it
5. You can also imagine your sit bones moving away from each other

It's important to do both long contractions as well as short quick contractions so the pelvic floor has all of its functions available when needed.

Long holds: Start with 5 sec and repeat 10 times. If you feel like you can do these fairly easily, then do a few sets or increase the time you're holding up to 10 sec for 10 times. Gradually work up to 2-3 times per day.

Short, quick squeezes: Squeeze quickly and then relax quickly 5 times in a row. If you can do those, you might increase to 10 times in a row. Gradually work up to 3 sets of these 2-3 times a day[50].

Pay attention to the range of motion you get from these contractions if you are able to feel them at all. If you can feel the range of motion, note how far it feels like it is going. As you continue these awareness exercises note if you feel as though the range of motion is increasing. If you cannot feel them yet, do not despair, keep at it as eventually the brain and body will make the connection to where you can feel the activation!

ABDOMINAL MUSCLE MOTION

Due to the main function of the abdominal muscles, it makes sense why you would want to be aware of them and how they function. In fact, you really need a high sense of awareness to properly activate them. This is done specifically through abdominal bracing. Abdominal bracing can be slight and nuanced. It can take time to learn how to do it correctly.

Muscle activation can be a bit tedious, but that's because we're actively building neural connections first[51]. Most know this as muscle memory. That memory has to come from somewhere and we can coax it along by thinking and imagining what we want that muscle to do.

ACTIVITY: Awareness of Abdominal Muscles

There are two types of awareness exercises you can choose from. One exercise is Partner Abdominal Awareness and the other is Individual Abdominal Awareness[52].

Partner Abdominal Awareness
1) Sit down in a chair or stand against a wall
2) Place your hands together in a prayer position and stick your arms straight out in front of you
3) Your partner should push against your hands trying to turn your body, resist that push
4) You should feel your abdominal muscle contract fairly easily
5) Have your partner push from each side, press up, then press down and pay attention to how your abdominals feel with each different type of force

Individual Abdominal Awareness
1) Stand up straight and tall against a wall or sit up very tall in a chair
2) Take your index and middle finger and place them on your sides where your waist is
3) Press your fingers gently into your sides
4) Begin to march in place and pay attention to what you feel underneath your fingers
5) If you are sitting, try and stand up, but keep at least one set of fingers on your side, pay attention to how that feels
6) If you are standing begin to walk around and make some abrupt stops or turns, pay attention to how that feels

You can also refer to the bracing exercises mentioned in Chapter 4 to give you two other methods for learning abdominal muscle awareness through bracing.

BACK MUSCLES

The muscles of the back are the main structural support for your trunk. They help you to move your body, arms, neck, head, shoulders, and your legs. The muscles of the back have such a far-reaching effect on how our body moves. This is mainly due to the attachment points of many of the muscles. For example; the latissimus dorsi attaches at the upper arm (if you lift your arm overhead, it creates the back edge of your armpit), the spine, and all the way down to the back upper edge of the pelvis. Other muscles go so far as to attach to the base of your skull, shoulder blade, and spine like the trapezius[53].

ACTIVITY: Awareness of Back Muscles

1) Sit tall in a chair or stand up tall
2) Place your hands on your waist with your fingers pointing backwards and thumbs pointing down
3) Brace or contract your abs and feel for your back muscles to contract as well
4) If you cannot feel these muscles, lightly cough and feel for a contraction
5) Pay close attention to how your back feels with an abdominal contraction or light coughing

Belly Breathing

Belly breathing is also referred to as diaphragmatic breathing or abdominal breathing. This type of breathing helps you to focus on breathing more with help from your diaphragm. This helps you breathe more efficiently and with less work. Diaphragmatic breathing has many benefits that can affect your entire body. It's the basis for many meditation and relaxation techniques, which can lower your stress levels and blood pressure, and regulate other critical bodily processes[54].

ACTIVITY: Diaphragmatic Breathing & Core Canister Breathing

The most basic type of diaphragmatic breathing is done by inhaling through your nose and breathing out through your mouth.

Diaphragmatic Breathing

Here's the basic procedure for diaphragmatic breathing. It may be easiest to practice while lying flat on your bed or the floor when you first start. You will want to practice this sitting down or standing up as well, given we don't live lives laying down all the time (it sure would be nice though).

1) Sit or lie down on a comfortable, flat surface
2) Relax your shoulders, shifting them downward away from the ears
3) Put a palm on your chest and a palm on your stomach
4) Inhale through your nose and allow your belly and chest to expand
5) Feel your rib cage expand to the sides and even through your back
6) Feel for your pelvic floor to expand away from you as well
7) Notice if you are "pushing" your belly or pelvic floor out. If so, try to avoid push and just ALLOW the natural expansion that happens with breathing.

<u>Core Canister Breathing</u>[55]
This method of breathing will give you awareness surrounding your core for breathing, when you add in the pelvic floor relaxation and activation, it will give you greater awareness in how your pelvic floor acts when you inhale and exhale along with your diaphragm.

Core Canister Method of Breathing: How to connect to your abdominal muscles, diaphragm, and pelvic floor.

- Inhalation – breathe wide into the ribcage and down into the abdomen
  - Diaphragm shortens and lowers to let the lungs expand
  - Abdominal wall expands as pressure increases with inhalation
  - Pelvic floor descends (intentionally relaxes) as intraabdominal pressure increases
- Exhalation – breath is coming up and out
  - Diaphragm relaxes as air moves out of the lungs
  - Abdominal wall contracts
  - Pelvic floor muscles contract

Core Connection Breath is when you add a more intentional pelvic floor contraction (or lift on the exhale breath)

Every one of these awareness exercises will serve you well if you take the time to practice them. The more aware you are of your body and how your muscles contract and relax the more control you will have over your movements. This means the better control you will have of your body in situations where you are moving with purpose and when you are not. Muscle memory and increased proprioception serves us most when we are moving without "thinking" about it, as this is when we are most likely to injure ourselves through a strained muscle or by losing our balance and falling. Remember, proprioception is how our body and brain communicate where our body is in space without us "telling" it. The better your brain and body can connect on where and how to move the better off nearly everything you do will be.

CHAPTER 7 - Core Stretching Exercises

Maintaining mobility as we age can be quite challenging. However, if you put in the work, the payoff is more than worth it and can dictate your quality of life and how much independence you have. The ligaments, tendons, muscles, and other soft tissues get less and less elastic, reducing mobility inherently as we age. This typically results in us moving and doing less, which compounds, leading to even more immobility. Stretching and exercise can help keep this from happening as fast, leaving you to enjoy more of your life.

A word on hypermobility. Just because you can doesn't mean you should. While joint hypermobility is very common (and kind of neat), it can cause issues. Hypermobility, also referred to as double-jointed, means your joints can move beyond the normal range of motion and that they are very flexible. The most commonly affected joints are your elbows, wrists, fingers and knees. If you are double-jointed, or hypermobile, you will want to practice restraint when stretching. Just because you can stretch to an excessive amount doesn't mean you should. In fact, you really shouldn't. When you stretch, you want to get to a point of tension and feel a slight pull or strain. Going farther really won't reap you any added benefits. Focus on gradual movements and not sudden or abrupt motions. Doing so may cause injury and a potential setback. One more word of caution when stretching, NEVER stretch a torn, bruised, or otherwise hurt muscle as it will only make the issue worse.

Additionally, some muscles that are overstretched and too loose, may feel "tight" and that's because they are not working properly. Stretching a loose muscle will not give you good results either. If you can't tell if you have a loose or injured muscle, check with your physician or a physical therapist to help you out.

How often should you stretch? How long should you hold a stretch? And how many times should you do each stretch? A panel of experts convened by the American College of Sports Medicine (ACSM) reviewed a wide range of studies to help answer these questions. Based on the evidence, the panel agreed that:

Healthy adults should do flexibility exercises (stretches, yoga, or tai chi) for all major muscle-tendon groups—neck, shoulders, chest, trunk, lower back, hips, legs, and ankles—at least two to three times a week. For optimal results, you should spend a total of 60 seconds on each stretching exercise[56].

The following stretches were chosen to be a part of a well-rounded flexibility program that will serve you best as you prepare to complete core strength exercises.

Aim for one to two sets holding at 60 seconds each.

Side Lying Spinal Twist

Stretches: tensor fascia lata (TFL), gluteus maximus, piriformis, shoulders, neck, internal/external obliques, erector spinae

Be careful if: you have a hernia, shoulder, knee, or hip replacement or injury

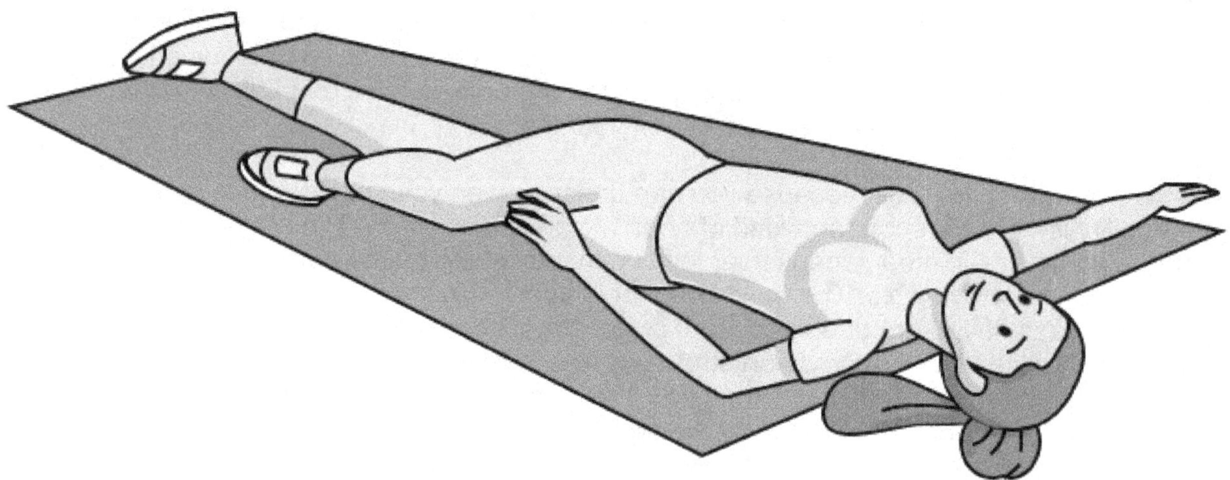

1. Lying on your back, bring your arms out to the sides with the palms facing down so that your body looks like the letter "T" from above.
2. Bend the right knee and place the right foot next to the left knee
3. Exhale drop the right knee over to the left side of your body, twisting the spine and low back. Look towards your right hand.
4. Keep the shoulders flat to the floor, close your eyes, and relax into the posture. Let gravity pull the knee down, so you do not have to use any effort in this posture
5. Breathe and hold for 6-12 breaths
6. To release: inhale and roll the hips back to the floor, exhale the leg back down to the floor, and repeat on the other side.

Modifications: Prioritize keeping your shoulders flat. If you feel like you need more support under your knees, feel free to place a folded blanket or foam roller underneath them. You can also bend both knees to make it a little easier to perform.

Variations: Press down on the knee that's stretching across your body. This additional weight will add to the stretch. You can also take very large, slow breaths to increase the stretch.

Corner Chest Stretch

Stretches: pectoralis major/minor, anterior deltoid, serratus anterior, coracobrachialis

Be careful if: you have issues with your neck, ribcage, shoulders, or chest

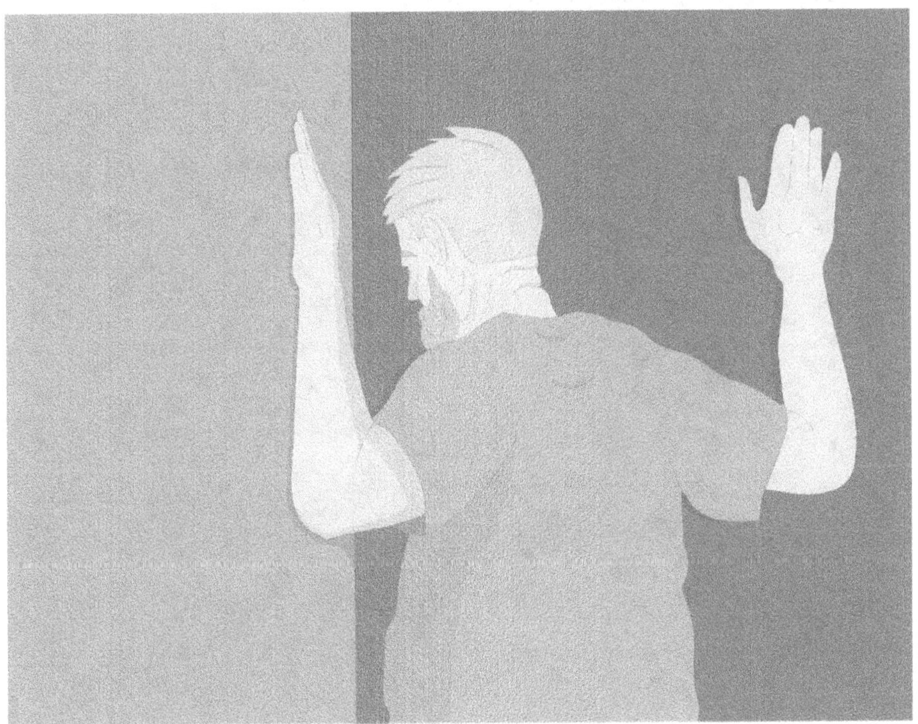

1. Stand facing the corner of a room
2.   With your palms facing the wall and elbows slightly below shoulder height, place each hand and forearm on each side of the corner
3. Inhale, then exhale and slowly lean into the stretch, think about bringing your entire torso toward the corner.
4. Keep your neck neutral and do not jut it out forwards
5. Breathe and hold for 6-12 breaths

Modifications: Sit in a chair and open your arms out wide to each side

Variations: Squeeze your shoulder blades together to increase the stretch

    Seated Doorway Chest Stretch
1. Sit upright in a sturdy chair, almost in the middle of a doorway
2. Place your hands on each side of the door frame and inhale
3. Exhale and bring your head and trunk as one segment forward until you feel a mild stretch in your chest
4. Breathe and hold for 6-12 breaths

Seated Calf Stretch

Stretches: calf (gastrocnemius, soleus), peroneals (or fibularis muscles), biceps femoris, semimembranosus

Be careful if: you have toe, foot, ankle, knee, or low back issues

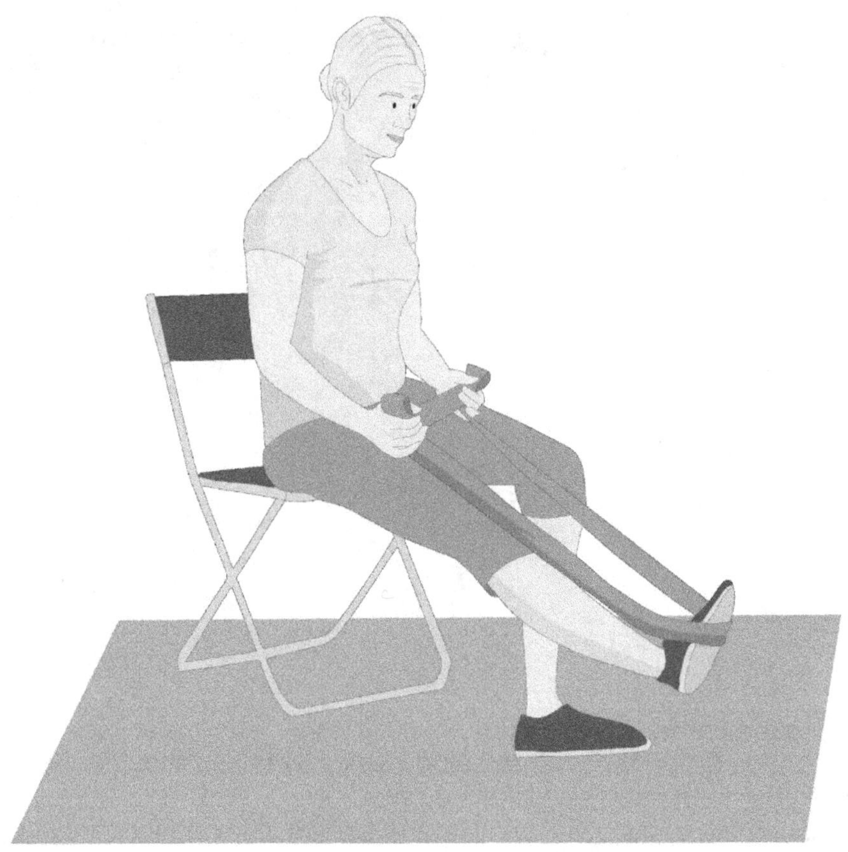

1. Sit upright in a sturdy chair about halfway forward on the seat
2. Keep your left leg bent and straighten out your right leg with the heel on the ground, toes pointing up
3. Loop a belt, towel, or exercise band around the ball of your right foot
4. Sitting up tall, breathe in
5. Exhale and lean forward from the hip and pulling the ball of your foot gently towards you, keeping your chest up
6. Breathe and hold for 6-12 breaths
7. Return to the starting position and repeat with the other foot

Modifications: Bend the knee of the outstretched leg or elevate the foot to make this a little easier.

Variations: Keeping your toes up, pivot your toes outward and inward to stretch more of the inner or outer aspect of your calf.

Seated Quadriceps Stretch

Stretches: quadriceps (rectus femoris, vastus lateralis/medialis/intermedius), hip flexors, psoas major/minor, iliacus, sartorius

Be careful if: you have ankle, knee, hip, or low back issues

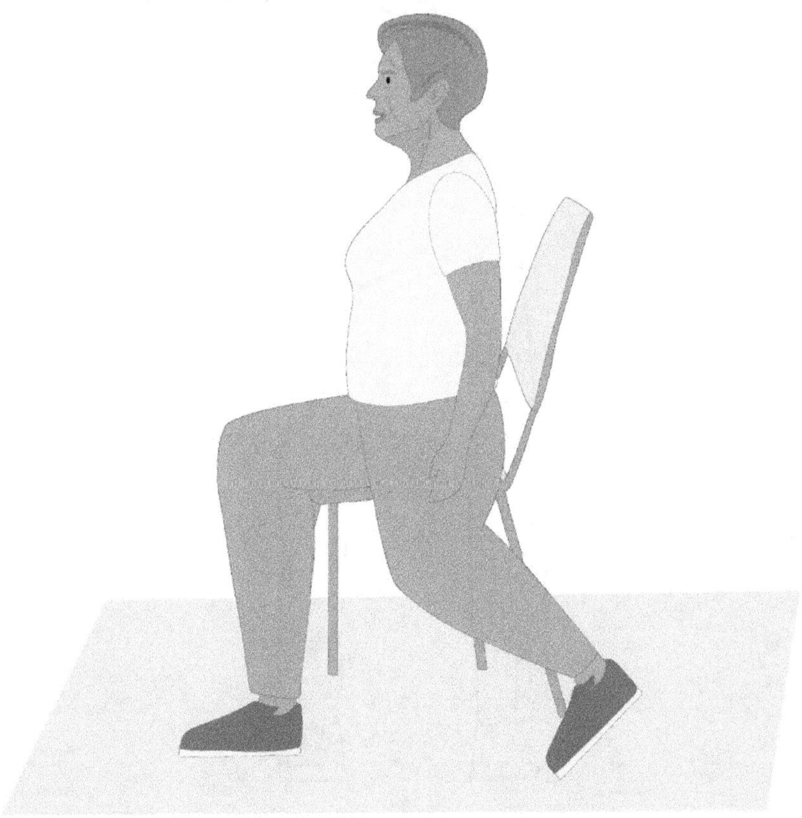

1. Sit upright in a sturdy chair
2. Scoot to the left until your left cheek is half off the chair, and hold onto something if you need to for balance.
3. Move the left foot back and let the left knee drop so it is pointing straight down at the ground.
4. Inhale and exhale as you stick your tailbone out backwards and lean back slightly
5. Breathe and hold for 6-12 breaths
6. Return to the starting position and repeat with the right leg

Modifications: Sit on a folded towel or a taller sturdy chair to decrease the amount of bending your knee has to do.

Variation: Twist away from the bent knee to increase the stretch or loop a belt around the ankle of the stretched leg and pull the foot back toward the buttock to increase the stretch

Upper Trapezius Stretch

Stretches: upper trapezius, sternocleidomastoid, scalenes, levator scapulae

Be careful if: you have neck, shoulder, thoracic spine (mid back), or wrist issues

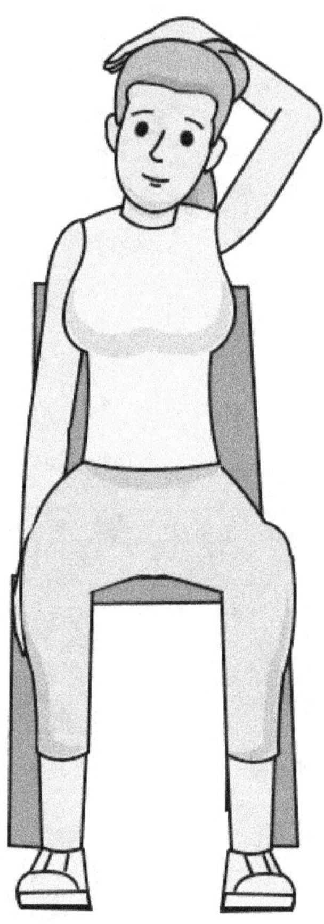

1. Sit upright in a sturdy chair or stand up tall
2. Eyes forward, tilt your head towards your left shoulder (don't bring your shoulder up to your ear, bring your head down to meet your shoulder).
3. Inhale and place your left hand on the right side of your head by reaching up and overhead.
4. Exhale and very gently draw the head towards the left shoulder
5. Reach towards the ground with your right hand to deepen the stretch.
6. Breathe and hold for 6-12 breaths
7. Return to the starting position and repeat on the other side.

Modifications: Shorten the stretch or don't pull with your hand.

Variation: For a deeper stretch, place the back of your right hand on your low back or mid back. You can also turn your gaze downward to the direction your head is tilted and change where you feel the stretch

Seated Hamstring Stretch

Stretches: hamstrings (biceps femoris, semitendinosus, semimembranosus), calf (gastrocnemius, soleus), adductors (inner thigh), erector spinae, gluteus maximus

Be careful if: you have any issues with the ankle, knee, hip, or low back issues

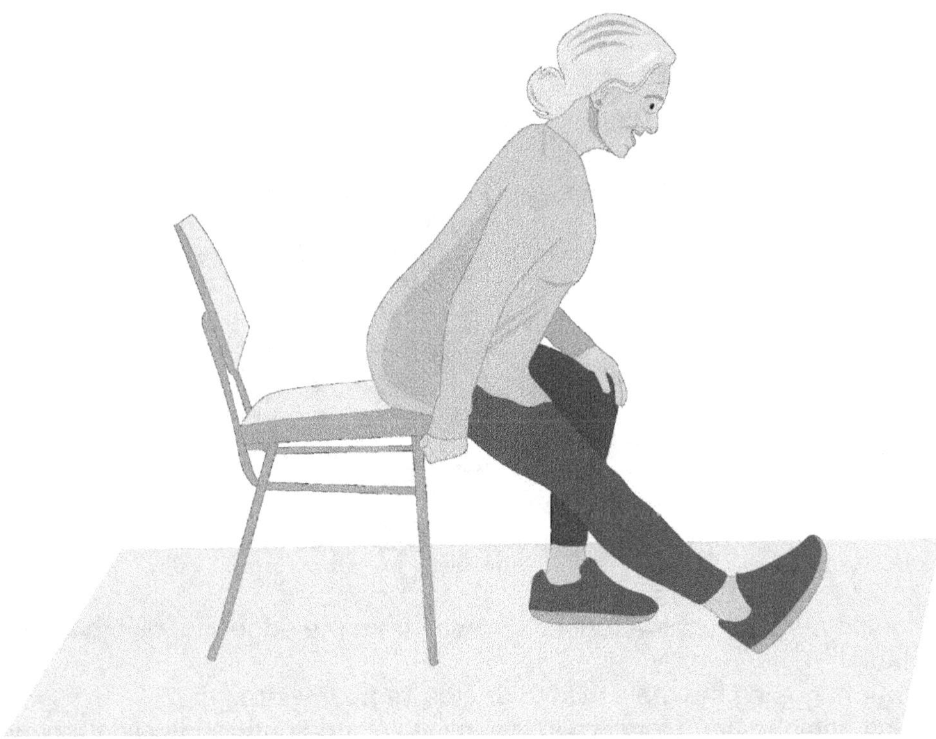

1. Sit upright in a sturdy chair about halfway forward on the seat
2. Keep your left leg bent and straighten out your right leg with the heel on the ground, toes pointing up
3. Sit up tall, breathe in, and raise your arms in front of you at shoulder height.
4. Exhale and lean slightly forward, hinging at the hips. Reach out in front of you but be sure to keep your chest up.
5. Breathe and hold for 6-12 breaths
6. Return to the starting position
7. Repeat with the other leg

Modifications: Bend the knee of the outstretched leg or prop the foot up on a yoga block or blanket to make this a little easier.

Variations: Use a towel, belt or exercise band and loop it around the arch of your foot to pull yourself into a deeper stretch. You can also flex the toe and straighten the leg for a deeper stretch.

Seated Table Lat Stretch

Stretches: latissimus dorsi, serratus anterior, teres major

Be careful if: you have elbow or shoulder issues or you cannot get your arms up overhead without pain and discomfort

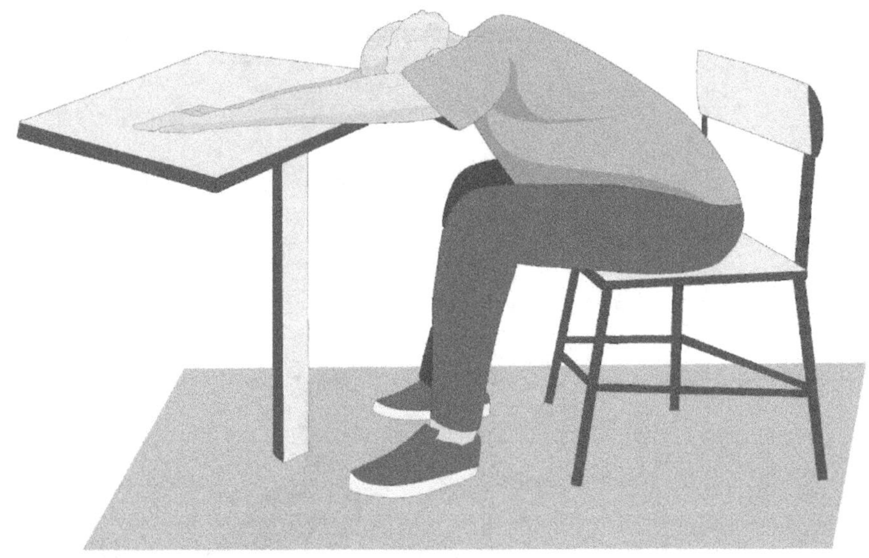

1. Sit upright in a sturdy chair a foot or so away from the edge of a dining table (not a coffee table)
2. Place your hands on the table with your elbows nearly straight
3. Inhale and begin to bend forward at the waist, letting your hands slide forward on the table
4. Exhale and continue to drop your chest towards the floor
5. Breathe and hold for 6-12 breaths

Modifications: Use a higher surface such as a countertop or bathroom vanity to make it a little easier

Variations: Place your arms on a foam roller or rolled-up towel to increase the stretch

Doorway Lat Stretch

1. Hold onto a door frame with your left hand so your left arm crosses over your body but remain standing in the doorway
2. Stagger your foot stance for balance
3. Inhale and begin to bend sideways to your right while pushing your left hip out and away
4. Exhale and sink into the stretch
5. Turn your pelvis towards the hand on the doorframe for a bigger stretch
6. Breathe and hold for 6-12 breaths

7. Return to the starting position and repeat with the other side

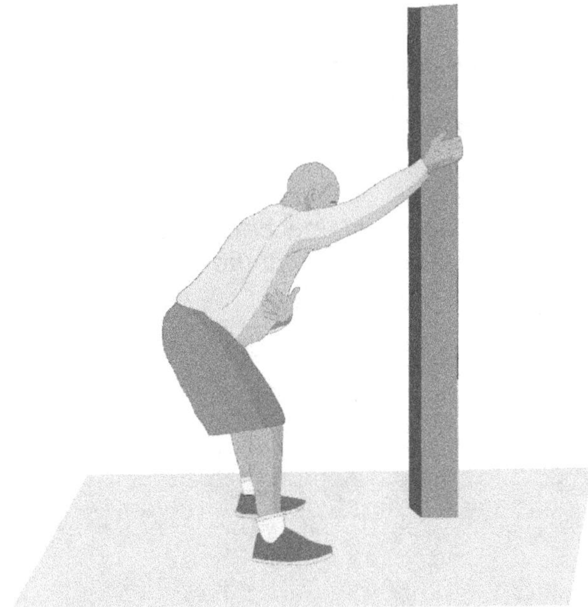

Wall Lat Stretch

1. Stand up straight and place your palms on a wall making sure your arms are straight
2. Inhale and begin to bend at the hip, keeping your hands where they are or letting them slide up the wall a bit
3. Exhale and drop your chest toward the ground
4. Breathe and hold for 6-12 breaths

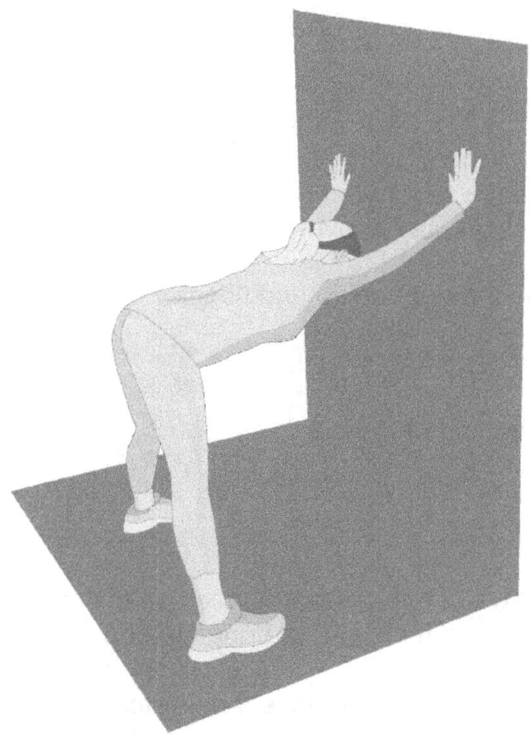

Seated Piriformis Stretch

Stretches: piriformis, gluteus maximus, superior/inferior gemellus, internal/external obturator, quadriceps femoris

Be careful if: you have sciatica or sciatic pain, low back or sacral issues, or hip replacement. If you have had a hip replacement, please use one of the modifications as this stretch may be too deep.

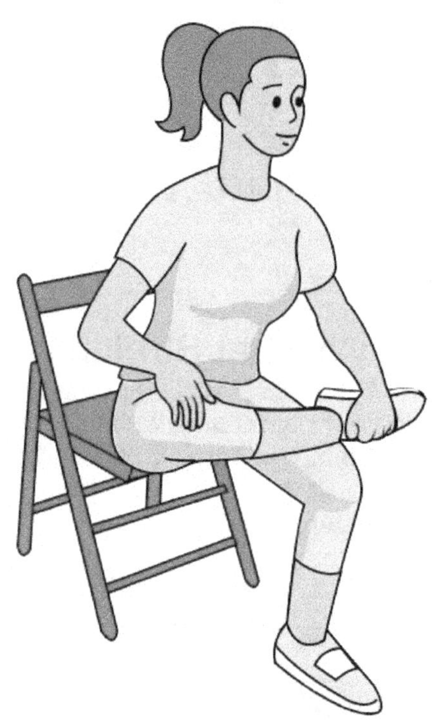

1. Sit upright in a sturdy chair about halfway forward on the seat
2. Place your right ankle on your left thigh, just above your knee so that your legs are making the number "4".
3. Place a hand on the right knee and the right ankle and flex the foot of your right leg so your toe is pointing forward.
4. Press gently into your right knee to begin the stretch.
5. Sitting up tall, breathe in
6. Exhale and lean slightly forward bending at the hip
7. Breathe and hold for 6-12 breaths
8. Return to the starting position
9. Repeat with the other leg

Modifications: Place a rolled-up blanket, towel, or yoga (foam) block on the inside of your left foot and rest the outer edge of your right foot on it instead of bringing it up to your knee.

Variations: Bring the foot closer to your hip crease to increase the stretch.

Seated Backbend

Stretches: rectus abdominis, external/internal oblique

Be careful if: you have low back, neck, or hip issues

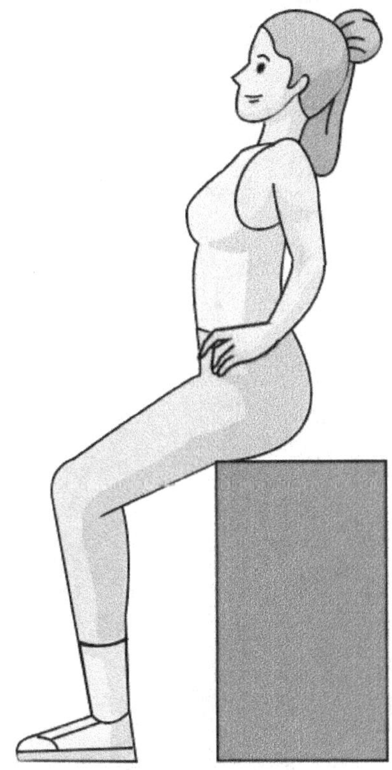

1. Sit upright in a sturdy chair about halfway forward on the seat
2. Place your hands on your lower back, knees, or hold on to the sides of the chair
3. Inhale and sit up tall
4. Exhale and begin to bend backwards slowly, going only as far as you are comfortable and able to remain breathing. Really focus on arching your back.
5. Breathe and hold for 6-12 breaths

Modifications: Before bending backwards, stick your tailbone out to increase the stretch without having to bend far as back

Variations: You can also perform this standing or bent backwards over a stability ball

Seated Overhead Stretch

Stretches: serratus anterior, rectus abdominis, external/internal obliques, latissimus dorsi, erector spinae

Be careful if: you have elbow, shoulder, or neck issues

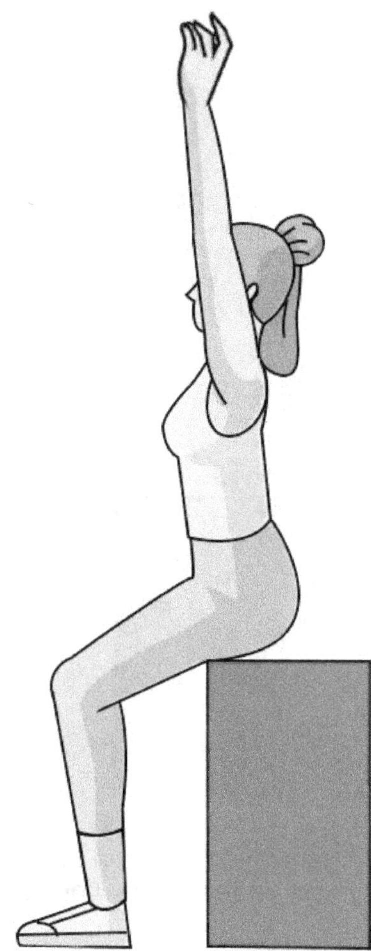

1. Sit upright in a sturdy chair about halfway forward on the seat
2. Reach your arms overhead, interlacing your fingers and inhale
3. Exhale and gently pull your extended overhead arms towards the back of the chair until you feel a stretch in your shoulders and sides
4. Breathe and hold for 6-12 breaths

Modifications: If you cannot raise your arms over your head, keep your arms down but draw the shoulders up and make them wide as though you are trying to make your stature large and wide like Frankenstein.

Variations: You can also hang from a bar or suspension trainer to increase the stretch

Seated Side Stretch

Stretches: intercostals (rib cage muscles), erector spinae, external/internal obliques, latissimus dorsi, quadratus lumborum, psoas

Be careful if: you have neck, shoulder, or ribcage issues

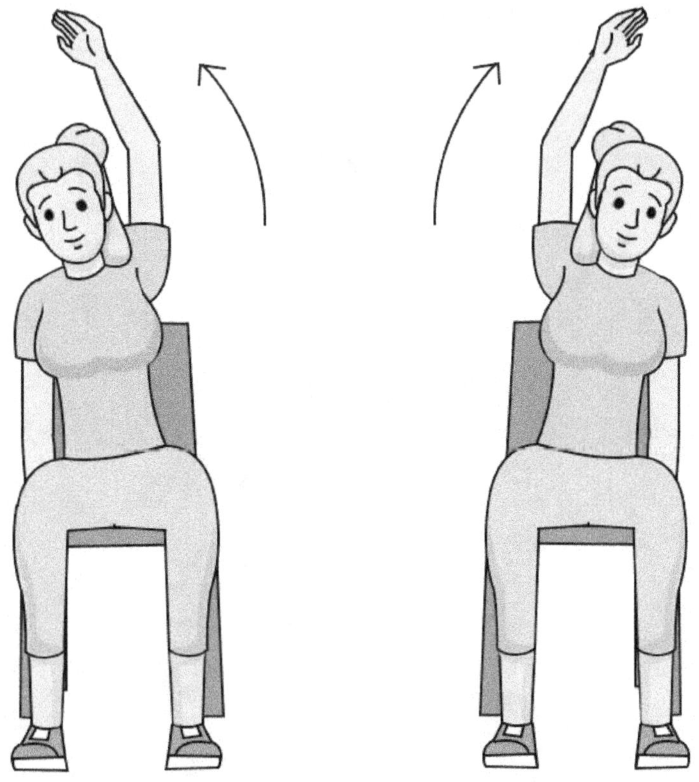

1. Sit upright in a sturdy chair about halfway forward on the seat
2. Reach your left arm up and inhale as you stretch the arm up high
3. Exhale and bend to the right, keeping your chest facing forward, with your left arm leaning to the right as you bend that way.
4. Breathe and hold for 6-12 breaths
5. Return to the starting position and repeat on the right side

Modifications: If you cannot raise your arms over your head, let your arm cross your body and draw the shoulder up and across, keeping your chest facing forwards. If you can reach an arm overhead but still feel unstable, place the opposite arm on a table or counter for stability.

Variations: Increase the stretch by reaching down to the ground with the opposite arm. You can also do this move standing.

Seated Triangle

Stretches: erector spinae, internal/external obliques, shoulders, hip flexors, adductors (inner thigh), neck

Be careful if: you have neck, shoulder, or low back issues

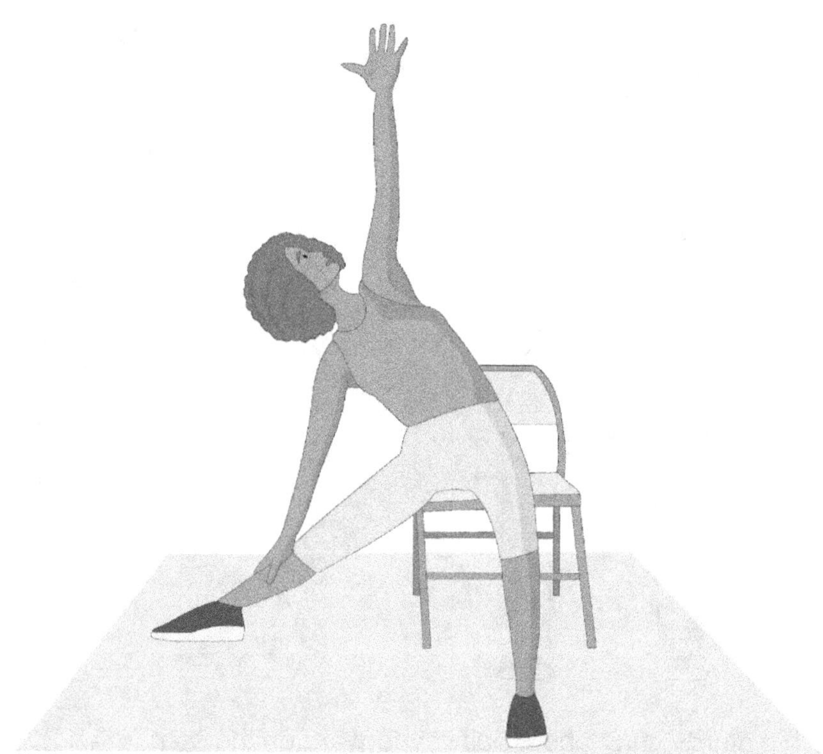

1. Sit upright in a sturdy chair, about halfway off the seat with your legs out wide
2. Place the back of your right forearm on the inside of your right thigh
3. Inhale and begin to bend forward at the hip letting the arm move towards the floor
4. Exhale and twist your trunk to left by bringing your left arm to point up towards the ceiling while the right one is pointing at or touching the ground
5. Turn your head up to look at your left hand
6. Breathe and hold for 6-12 breaths
7. Slowly return to the starting position and switch sides

Seated Butterfly Stretch

Stretches: adductors (inner thigh), hamstrings, tensor fascia lata (TFL)

Be careful if: you have groin or knee issues, or have had a hip replacement

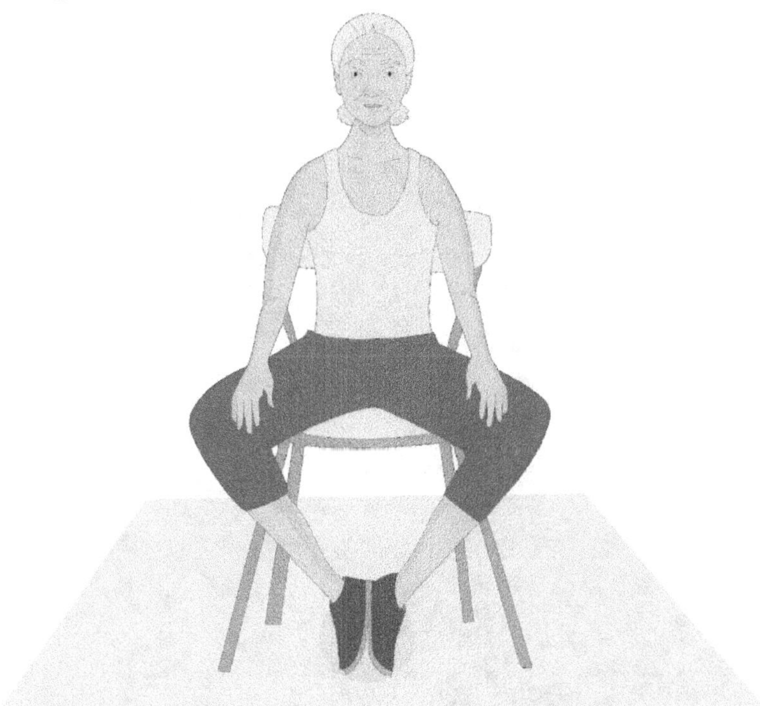

1. Sit upright in a sturdy chair about halfway forward on the seat
2. Place your feet together side-by-side and let your knees fall out wide.
3. Inhale and place your hands on the inside of your knees
4. Exhale, bend forward a bit at the waist and gently press your knees outward
5. Breathe and hold for 6-12 breaths

Modifications: Widen the feet or sit on a rolled-up towel or taller chair to make this stretch easier.

Variations: Bring the feet up higher to increase the stretch, you can also press your knees down and to the outside to increase the stretch

Trapezius and Hamstring Combination

Stretches: hamstrings (biceps femoris, semitendinosus, semimembranosus), upper trapezius, erector spinae, gluteus maximus

Be careful if: you have neck, shoulder, thoracic spine (mid back), wrist, ankle, knee, hip, or low back issues

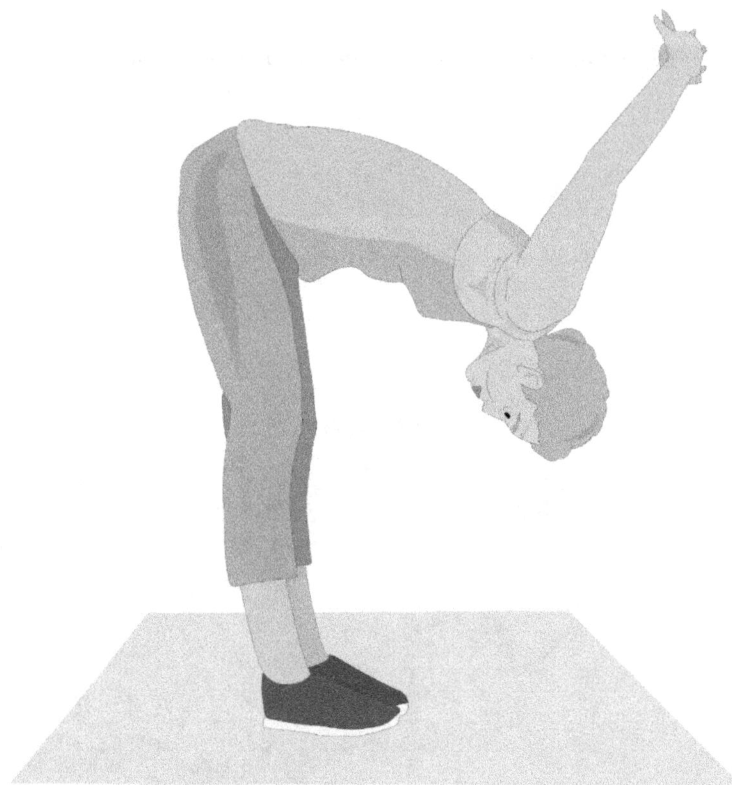

1) Stand with your feet shoulder-width apart and your knees slightly bent.
   a) You can stand against a wall for stability.
2) Hold your arms behind your back, interlocking your fingers.
3) Slowly bend forward at the waist, keeping your back straight.
4) As you bend forward, lift your arms up behind you as high as you comfortably can.
5) Breathe and hold for 6-12 breaths
6) Rise slowly so you don't make yourself dizzy

One of the "breaks" we get with flexibility, mobility, and strength training is it doesn't necessarily need to be done all at once. Stretching, especially, takes time, and you may not have the time to perform every stretch on the days you choose to do them. You can split stretches up throughout the day or week, depending on the kind of time you have. If you can get them all in at once, great! However, if you cannot, you have the option to structure it in a way that works best for you!

Stretching is one of the most effective ways to keep pain at bay, remain strong, maintain good blood circulation, and stay mobile and independent, among other things. Not only that, your balance and stability are dependent on the mobility of your body, namely your lower body. Stretching can also help you to maintain doing things like tying your shoes, picking things up off of the ground, brushing or washing your hair, putting on clothes, scratching your back, cooking and cleaning, stooping down to garden, and many other daily tasks!

CHAPTER 8 - Mat & Floor Core Exercises

Probably the most familiar of core strength exercises are those done from the floor. Just the act of getting down onto the floor, performing one of these exercises, and returning to a standing position activates nearly the entirety of your core musculature. Additionally, gravity will play a prominent role in making these exercises more challenging. The goal is to utilize your body weight, gravity, and a safe amount of instability to push your body to use some ab muscles that, for some of us, might not have been utilized for quite a while. All of these obstacles together will help you see greater and potentially faster benefits.

That being said, take these exercises with a grain of salt and pay attention to how your body feels during each. Some may be too challenging or just not feel right, while others may help you focus on and activate specific target muscles. It's okay to pick and choose which are best for you. As we begin, move slowly and purposefully to minimize risk of injury and try not to use momentum in these movements. Feel free to perform your own variation or use assistance as well. We're here to meet you wherever you are in your fitness journey.

If you already follow a strength routine but don't specifically focus on core work, try adding 2 or 3 these exercises a few times per week (Harvard Health Publishing, 2023). Bear in mind that extra core strength work will likely fatigue larger muscle groups and can impact your other training goals. Try it for a few weeks, but feel free to integrate core strength into your workouts however works best for you.

Perform one to three sets of each exercise you choose. Aim for 12-15 quality repetitions of each. You can break these repetitions up if you need to, or make the repetition range a goal.

PLANKS

A somewhat new tried and true style of core strengthening; planks are an anti-flexion movement. This means they will help keep your spine from bending too far forward, which helps keep your spine strong for actions that require bending forward to pick something up off the ground or so you can bend backward and stay stable.

When performing a plank, keep your core engaged, maintain a neutral spine, and be sure to breathe. This will help you perform the plank correctly and target the correct muscles[58]

Forearm Plank

Works: rectus abdominis, external/internal obliques, transverse abdominis, erector spinae, trapezius, latissimus dorsi, pectorals (chest muscles), serratus anterior, deltoids, biceps, triceps, glutes, hamstrings, and quads

Be careful if: You have shoulder, elbow, neck, low-, mid-, low-back, knee or hip issues

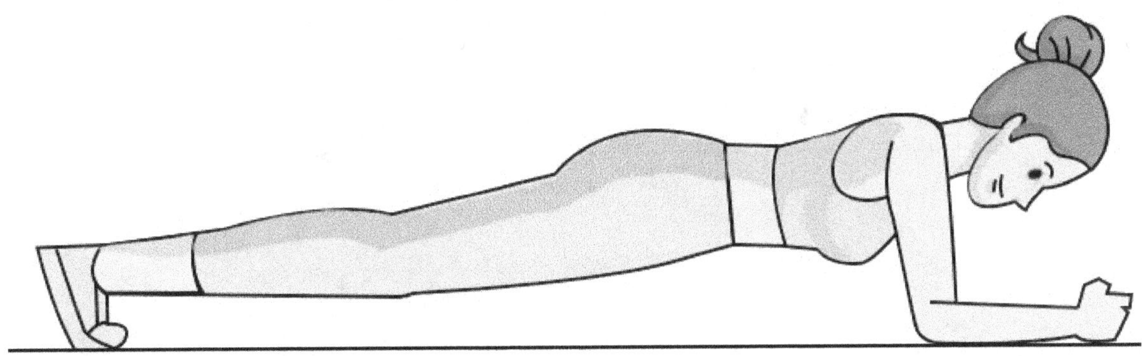

1) Lay on your stomach with your elbows and forearms at your side, palms down
2) Your elbows should be stacked underneath your shoulders
3) Inhale, contract your core and glutes (perform a pelvic tilt) and lift your body off the ground by pressing into your forearms and toes
4) Maintain a neutral spine and neck by looking a foot in front of you and keep your tailbone tucked so your hips do not sag or poke up too far
   a) It's called a plank because you should be straight as a board from the back of your head to your toes
5) Hold this position for as long as you can maintain proper form, up to 60 seconds

Make it easier: bring one or both knees down

Make it harder: come up on to your hands, lift one foot off the ground, lift one hand off the ground, rock your hips gently from side to side

Side Plank with Rotation

Works: external/internal obliques, transverse abdominis, erector spinae, trapezius, latissimus dorsi, serratus anterior, rotator cuff muscles, gluteus medius

Be careful if: You have shoulder, neck, low-, mid-, low-back, knee or hip issues.

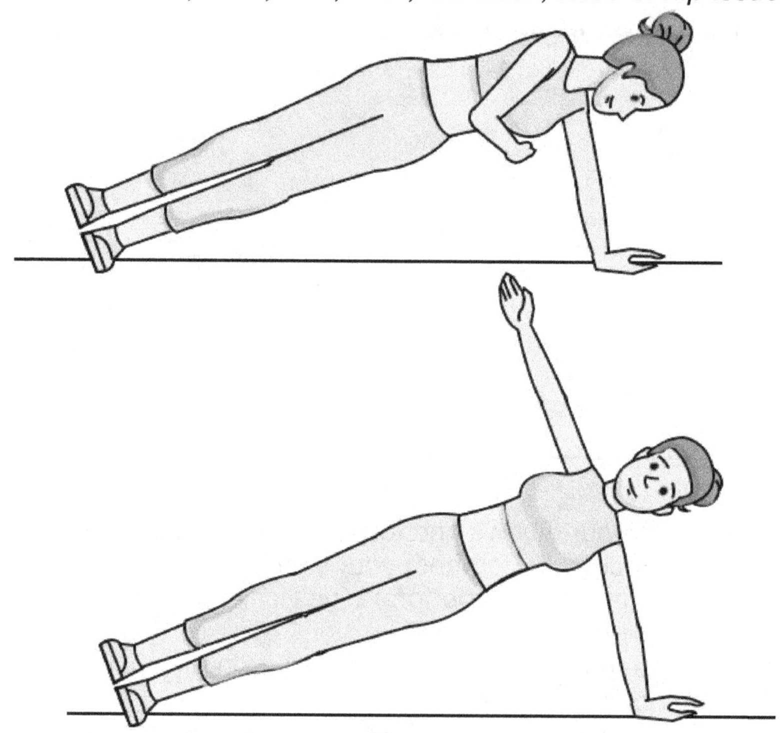

1) Lie on your right side with your legs straight and your feet stacked on top of one another or one in front of the other
2) Place your forearm flat on the ground, the elbow should be stacked under your shoulder
3) Inhale, contract your core and glutes (perform a pelvic tilt) and lift your hips up off the ground by pressing into your forearm and feet
4) Your head, shoulders, hips, knees, and feet should all be in line together
5) Maintain a neutral spine and neck by looking straight ahead of you and keep your tailbone tucked so your hips do not poke back too far
6) Slowly extend your top arm up to the ceiling and then dive it down in front of you, reaching between the floor and your ribcage.
    a) Your top shoulder will roll forward, and your mid-back will twist a bit
    b) Note: Think about reaching underneath your body to grab a marble.

Make it easier: Don't rotate as far or leave the arm up toward the ceiling

Make it harder: Perform the arm dive more slowly, use a small hand weight or exercise band

Side Plank

Works: external/internal obliques, transverse abdominis, erector spinae, trapezius, latissimus dorsi, serratus anterior, rotator cuff muscles, glutes

Be careful if: You have shoulder, neck, low-, mid-, low-back, knee or hip issues

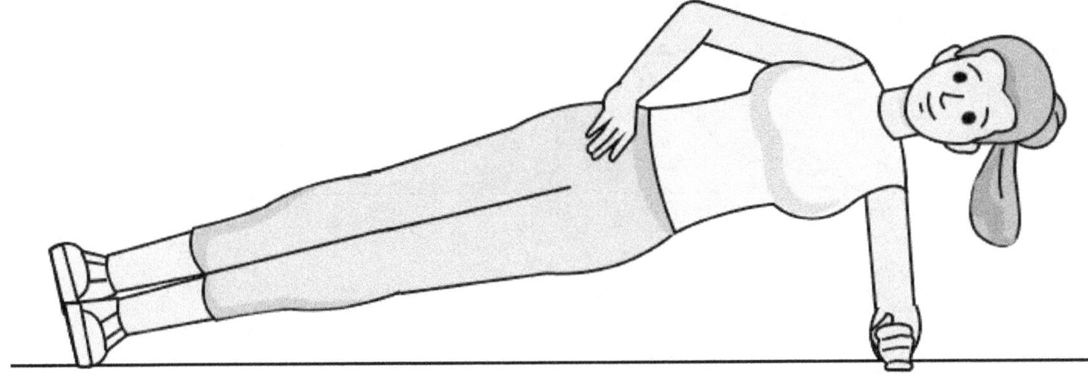

1. Lie on your right side with your legs straight and your feet stacked on top of one another or one in front of the other
2. Place your forearm flat on the ground, the elbow should be stacked under your shoulder
3. Inhale, contract your core and glutes (perform a pelvic tilt) and lift your hips up off the ground by pressing into your forearm and feet
4. Your head, shoulders, hips, knees and feet should all be in-line together
5. Maintain a neutral spine and neck by looking straight ahead of you and keep your tailbone tucked so your hips do not poke back too far
6. Hold this position for as long as you can maintain proper form, up to 60 seconds

Make it easier: Widen how far apart your feet are, bring one or both knees down, perform with your back against a wall to maintain good form

Make it harder: Come up on to your hand, lift top leg up

CRUNCHES AND CURL UPS

These are the traditional core strength exercises that we all know so well. They aren't for everyone, but they are tried and true! These types of activities focus on the "6-pack" muscles (*rectus abdominis*) mainly.

Crunch

Works: rectus abdominis, erector spinae, transverse abdominis, external/internal obliques

Be careful if: You have neck, mid-, or lower back issues

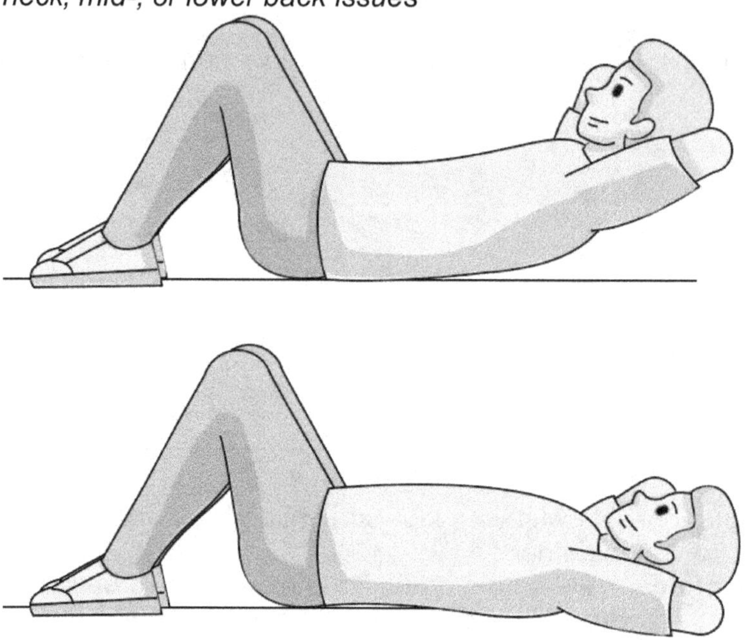

1) Lay down on the floor or a mat
2) Bend your knees so they point towards the ceiling, feet flat on the floor
3) Place a rolled-up towel, blanket or foam roller underneath your lower back for support
   a) You can place your hands on your belly, to your side, or gently behind your head but don't pull on your neck
4) Inhale and press your lower back into the towel.
5) Slowly peel your spine away from the floor, vertebrae by vertebrae until you are about halfway up. Focus on really engaging the core. Then exhale slowly. Maintain a forward gaze to ensure a neutral neck.
6) Hold for 1-3 seconds and return to the floor vertebrae by vertebrae

Make it easier: Hold for less time, curl up less, lie on an incline bench, extend both legs or one leg so it's rest on the ground

Make it harder: Bring feet off of the ground (held off the floor), bring knees to a 90-degree angle, hold the curl for up to 10 seconds or perform sitting on a folded-up towel or balance pad.

Single Leg Reverse Crunch

Works: rectus abdominis, transverse abdominis, external/internal obliques, quadratus lumborum, erector spinae, hip flexors

Be careful if: You have neck, mid-, or lower back issues

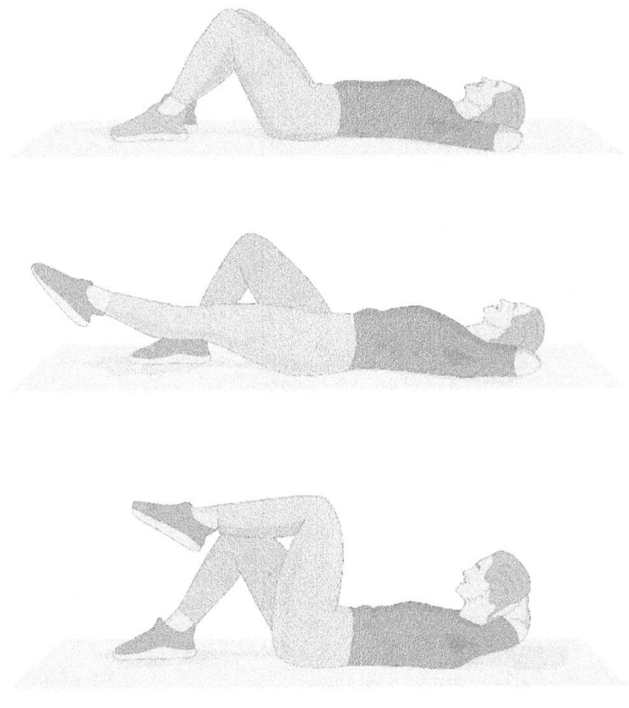

1) Lay down on the floor or a mat
2) Bend your left knee so it points toward the ceiling, foot flat on the floor
3) Keep your right leg extended or bend the knee slightly
4) Place a rolled-up towel (or similar) underneath your lower back for support
   a) You can place your hands on your belly, to your side, or behind your head, but don't pull on your neck
5) Inhale and press your lower back into the towel
6) Slowly peel your upper spine away from the floor vertebrae by vertebrae, exhaling slowly, and bring the knee of your right leg towards your head while keeping your left foot planted on the floor.
7) Maintain a forward gaze to ensure a neutral neck. Hold for 1-2 seconds.
8) Return to the floor vertebrae by vertebrae
9) Switch legs and repeat

Make it easier: Curl up less, don't bring the knee as high up

Make it harder: Hold the curl for up to 10 seconds, raise your arms overhead or out to your sides, lie on a decline bench

Reverse Crunch

Works: rectus abdominis, transverse abdominis, external/internal oblique, hip flexors

Be careful if: You have low back issues

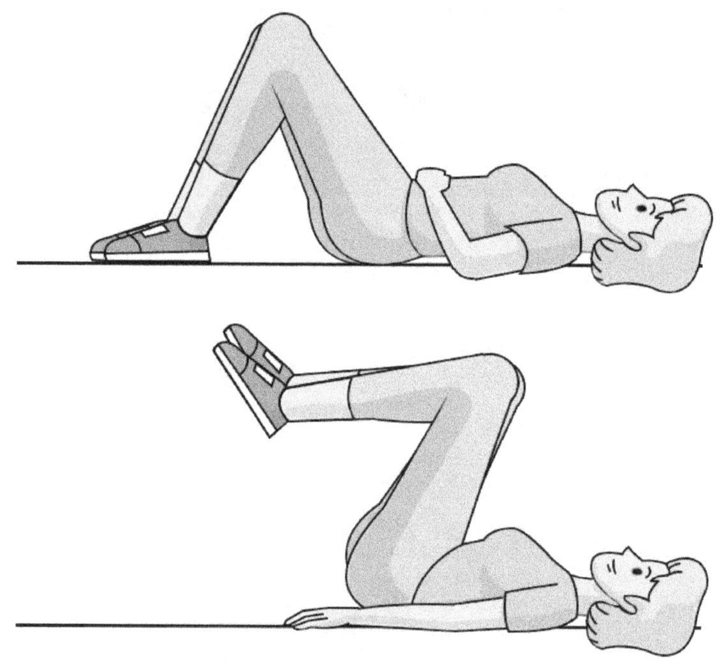

1) Lay down on the floor or a mat.
2) Bend both knees so they point toward the ceiling, feet flat on the floor.
3) Place a rolled-up towel (or similar) underneath your lower back for support
   a) You can place your hands on your belly, to your side, or behind your head, but don't pull on your neck
4) Inhale and press your lower back into the towel
5) Slowly pull your knees towards your chest until they're at a 90-degree angle, hips may come off the ground, exhaling slowly
   a) Note: This is called a reverse crunch because your lower body is moving rather than crunching up with your upper body.
6) Hold for 1-3 seconds
7) Return to the floor vertebrae by vertebrae

Make it easier: Don't bring the knees as far up, elevate your hips a bit for a shorter range of motion, bend the knee more.

Make it harder: Curl up more slowly, hold the curl for up to 10 seconds, straighten the legs more, lie on an incline bench

Bicycle Crunch

Muscles worked: external/internal obliques, rectus abdominis, transverse abdominis, hip flexors, quadriceps, hamstrings

Be careful if: You have hip, low-, or mid-back issues

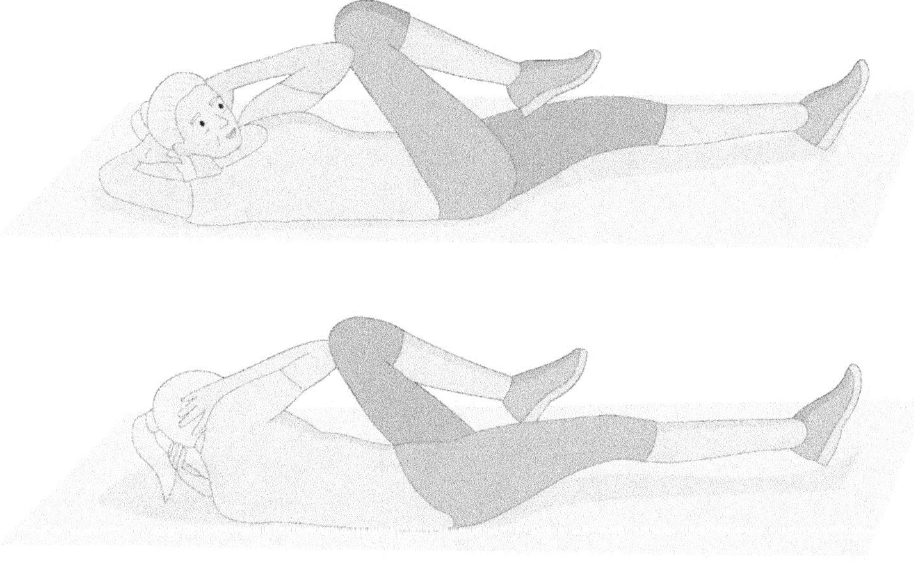

1) Lay down on the floor or a mat
2) Bend your knees so they point towards the ceiling
3) Place a rolled-up towel (or similar) underneath your lower back for support
   a) Place each hand next to or behind the ears, but do not pull on your neck.
   b) You can clasp them behind your head as well
4) Inhale and press your lower back into the towel
5) Slowly pull your left knee towards your head and reach your right elbow across your torso and towards the left knee, while extending your right leg, exhaling slowly
   a) The elbow and knee do not have to touch, get them as close together as you can without pain or discomfort
6) Hold for 1-3 seconds
7) Lower slowly, switch sides, and repeat

Make it easier: Perform the knee and elbow cross separately, leave one leg extended, reach with your hand instead of your elbow

Make it harder: Keep both legs off of the ground, touch the elbow to the knee, hold for up to 10 seconds, straighten your leg to start

Oblique Crunch (also Diagonal Crunch)

Works: external/internal oblique, hip flexors

Be careful if: You have neck, mid-, or lower back issues

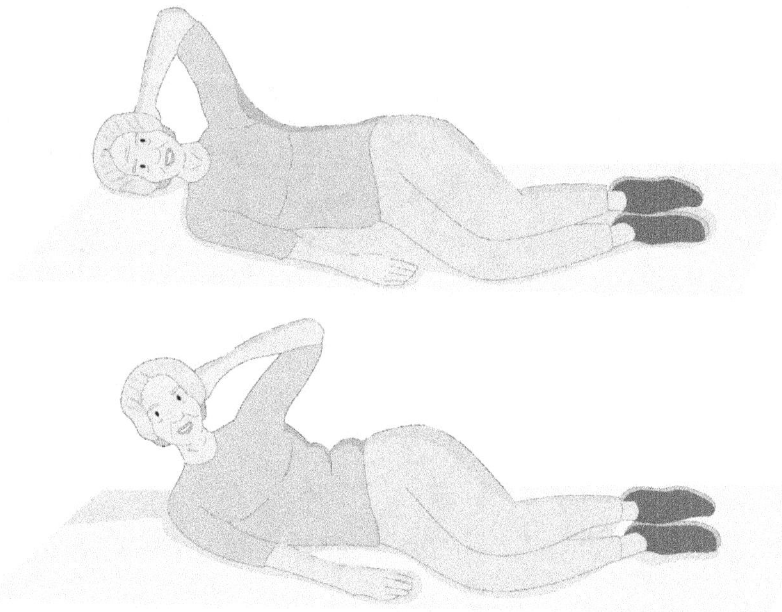

1) Lay down on a floor or mat on your right side, shoulders and hips aligned, knees slightly in front of your body.
   a) Bend your knees so your feet are behind you and can act as a stabilizer
2) Place your right arm underneath your head, your left hand can rest on your side.
3) Squeeze your glutes a bit (perform a pelvic tilt) and inhale.
4) Slowly bring your right side off of the ground as far as you comfortably can, exhaling slowly. Think of this as a twisted variation of a crunch that focused mainly on working the obliques.
5) Hold for 1-3 seconds
6) Slowly return to the floor
7) Switch sides and repeat

Make it easier: Don't come up as far, lie on an incline bench, use your top arm to help assist you in the movement by pushing into the floor and lifting the upper body off the ground

Make it harder: Come up more slowly, hold the curl for up to 10 seconds, lie on a decline bench, perform on a stability ball

Sit Up

Works: rectus abdominis, transverse abdominis, external/internal oblique, hip flexors

Be careful if: You have neck, mid-, or lower back issues

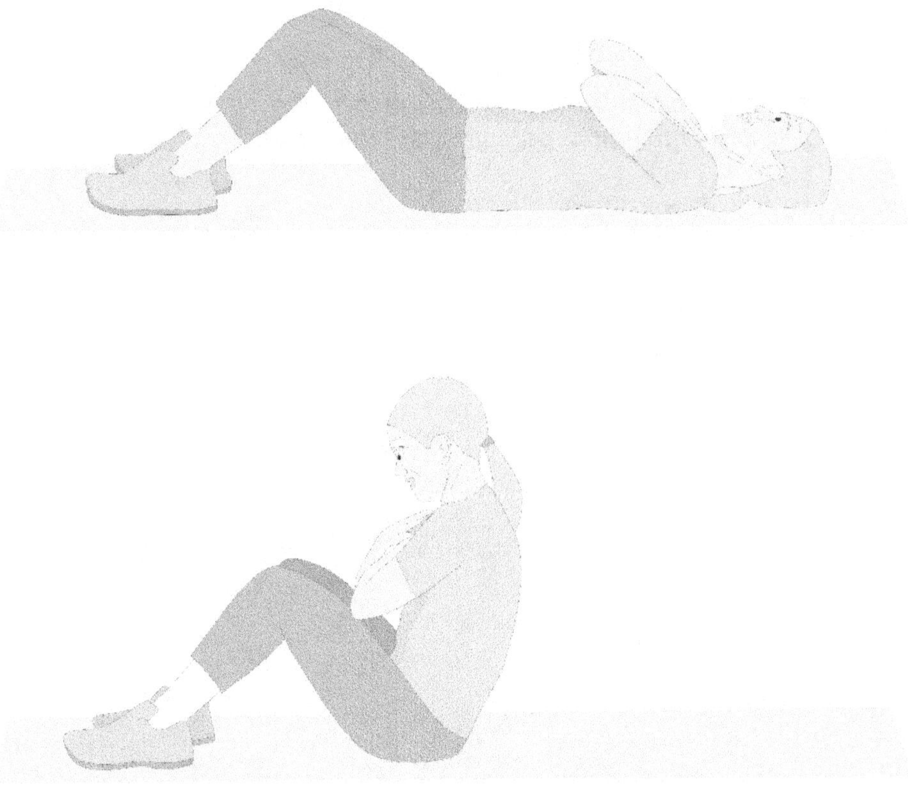

1) Lay down on the floor or a mat
2) Bend your knees so they point toward the ceiling, feet flat on the floor
3) Place a rolled-up towel (or similar) underneath your lower back for support
   a) You can place your hands on your belly, to your side, or behind your head, but don't pull on your neck
4) Inhale and press your lower back into the towel
5) Slowly peel your spine away from the floor vertebrae by vertebrae, exhaling slowly bringing your back off the floor as far as you comfortably can
6) Maintain a forward gaze to ensure a neutral neck
7) Hold for 1-3 seconds
8) Return to the floor vertebrae by vertebrae

Make it easier: Don't come up as far, lie on an incline bench, hold on to the front of your knees or back of your thighs, use a belt or exercise band looped behind your knee

Make it harder: Curl up more slowly, hold the curl for up to 10 seconds, lie on a decline bench, perform on a stability ball

SUPINE (lying face up) EXERCISES

Crunches and sit-ups aren't the only core strengthening exercises you can perform while laying on your back. There are a ton of different ways you can move your body and target your core musculature. Supine exercises are a great addition to any core strengthening program. These types of exercises will help to train the spinal stabilizers to resist too much flexion or backward motion at the spine. This can help you maintain good posture while standing, coming back from bending forward, or allow you to more safely bend backward at the waist.

Supine Toe Taps

Muscles worked: rectus abdominis, transverse abdominis, erector spinae, external/internal obliques, quadriceps, gluteus maximus, hamstrings, hip flexors

Be careful if: You have hip issues

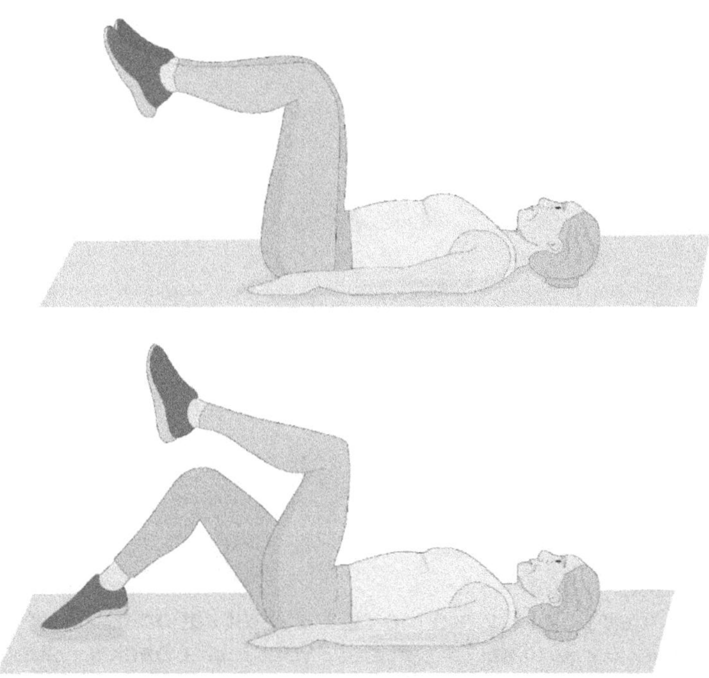

1. Lay down on the floor or a mat
2. Bend your knees so they point towards the ceiling, feet should be flat on the floor
3. Place your hands, palm down, on the floor next to you
4. Place a rolled-up towel (or similar) underneath your lower back for support
5. Inhale and press your lower back into the towel
6. Lift both legs off of the ground until your thighs are perpendicular to the ceiling (90-degree angle)
7. Drop your right leg slowly to the ground to a count of 3-5, exhaling slowly
8. Tap the toe of your right foot to the ground and return to start
9. Switch legs and repeat with the left leg

Make it easier: Don't let the foot go down so low, bend the knees more, leave one leg down

Make it harder: Drop the foot for up to 10 seconds, bring your shoulders up off the ground, straighten your legs more

Single Leg Abdominal Press

Muscles worked: transverse abdominis, external/internal obliques, quadriceps, hip flexors

Be careful if: You have low back, knee, or shoulder issues

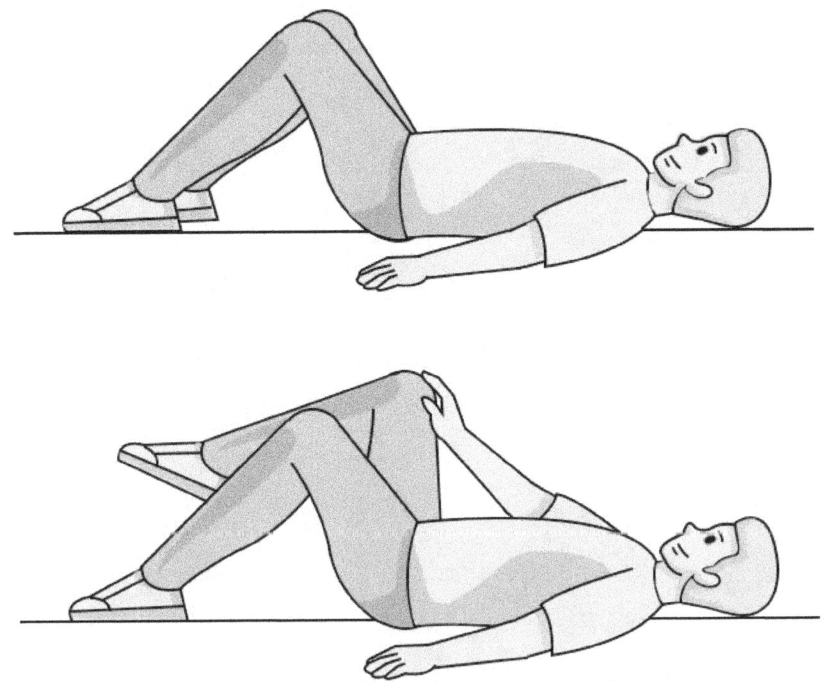

1) Lay down on the floor or a mat
2) Bend your left knee so it points towards the ceiling, foot should be flat on the floor
3) Keep your right leg extended or bend the knee slightly
4) Place a rolled-up towel (or similar) underneath your lower back for support
    a) You can place your hands on your belly, to your side, or behind your head but don't pull on your neck
5) Inhale and press your lower back into the towel
6) Extend your right hand towards your right knee as you bring it up towards you. Focusing on using your abs to lift your leg up and towards you.
7) Press your knee into your hand and hold for 3-5 seconds
    a) You can also press the knee out or in for some variation

Make it easier: Elevate the foot on the ground

Make it harder: Keep opposite leg off of the ground, hold for up to 10 seconds, bring your shoulders up off the ground

Lying Pelvic Tilt (Anterior & Posterior)

Muscles worked: quadriceps, erector spinae, multifidus, quadratus lumborum, external/internal oblique, psoas (anterior), hamstring, quadriceps, gluteus maximus/medius, rectus abdominis, external/internal oblique (posterior)

Be careful if: You have low back issues

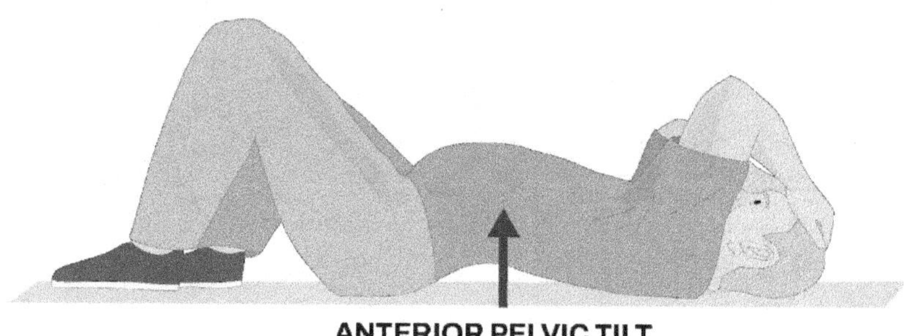

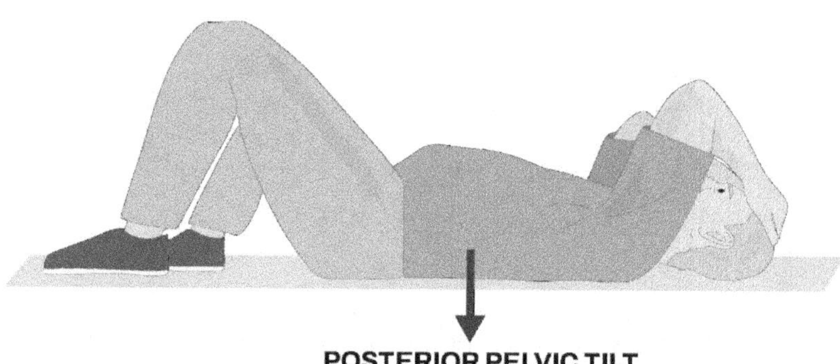

1. Lay on the floor or a mat with your knees up and feet flat on the floor
2. Place your hands on your hips or on the floor next to you

(Posterior Pelvic Tilt)
3. Inhale and slowly rock the top of your hips back and tuck your tailbone under, you'll feel your lower back pressing into the floor
4. Hold for 1-3 seconds, exhaling slowly

(Anterior Pelvic Tilt)
5. Inhale and begin to reverse this motion
6. Exhale slowly and begin to stick your tailbone "out" or towards the floor
7. Hold for 1-3 seconds

Make it easier: Put a towel between your low back and the floor for more feedback as to how your pelvis is moving

Make it harder: Elevate your feet for larger range of motion

Butterfly Crunch

Muscles worked: *rectus abdominis, transverse abdominis, erector spinae, external/internal obliques, hip flexors, adductors*

Be careful if: *You have knee, groin, or hip issues*

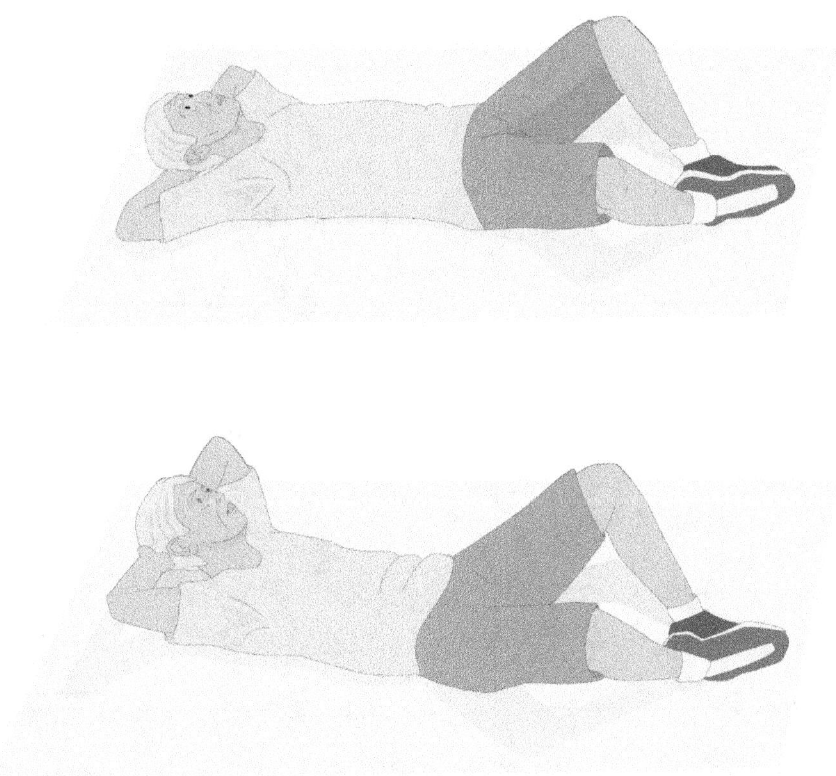

1) Lay on the floor or a mat with your knees up and feet flat on the floor
2) Place a rolled-up towel under your lower back
3) Inhale, brace your core, press into the towel
    a) You can place your hands on your belly, to your side, or behind your head but don't pull on your neck
4) Drop your knees open (place something on either side if you need to for support)
5) Exhale slowly and curl your vertebrae up one by one as far as you can comfortably go. Think of this as a regular crunch but with your knees out to the side.
6) Hold for 1-3 seconds
7) Slowly lower back down to the floor vertebrae by vertebrae

Make it easier: *Don't curl up as far, lay on an incline bench, straighten one leg*

Make it harder: *Hold for up to 10 seconds, bring legs up when you curl forward*

Glute Bridge

Muscles worked: gluteus maximus/medius, external/internal obliques, rectus abdominis, transverse abdominis, adductors, erector spinae

Be careful if: You have ankle, knee, or hip issues

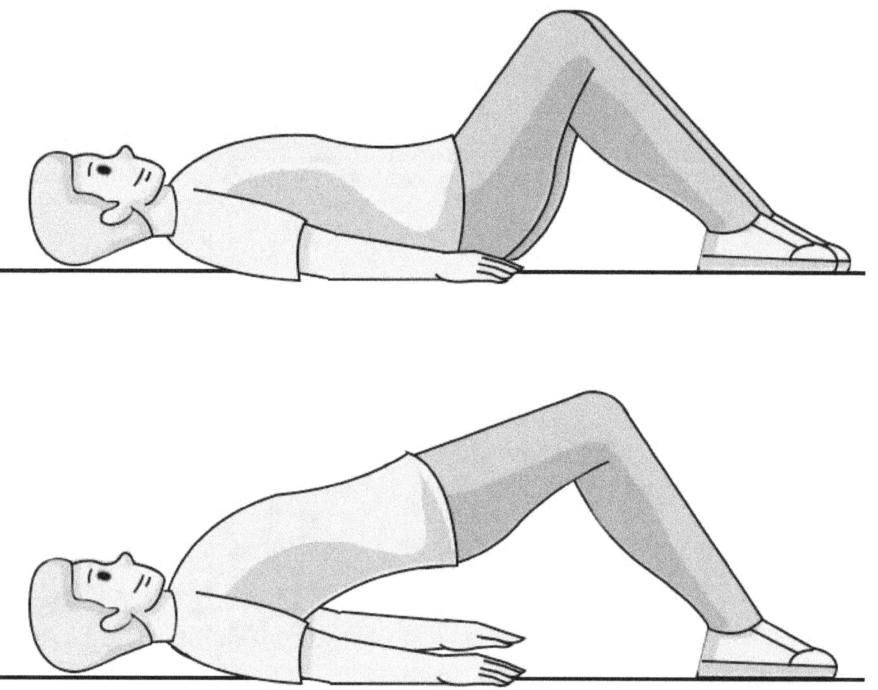

1) Lay down on the floor or a mat with your legs bent, feet flat on the floor
2) Place a rolled-up towel (or similar) underneath your lower back for support
3) Place each hand next to or behind the ears but do not pull on your neck
    a) You can clasp them behind your head as well
4) Inhale and press your lower back into the towel and tuck the chin a bit
5) Press into both feet (focus on pressing through the heels) and squeeze your glutes to bring your hips up off of the floor, exhaling slowly
    a) Your aim is to create a flat surface from shoulders to knees, avoid excessive inward curvature of the low back
6) Hold for 1-3 seconds, relax and return to start

Make is easier: Don't lift your hips as high

Make it harder: Elevate your feet, hold for up to 10 seconds, hold a dumbbell or barbell across your hips, perform with one leg, perform a march while hips are up.

Heel Touches (also Side Heel Taps)

Muscles worked: external/internal obliques, rectus abdominis, transverse abdominis

Be careful if: You have low-back issues

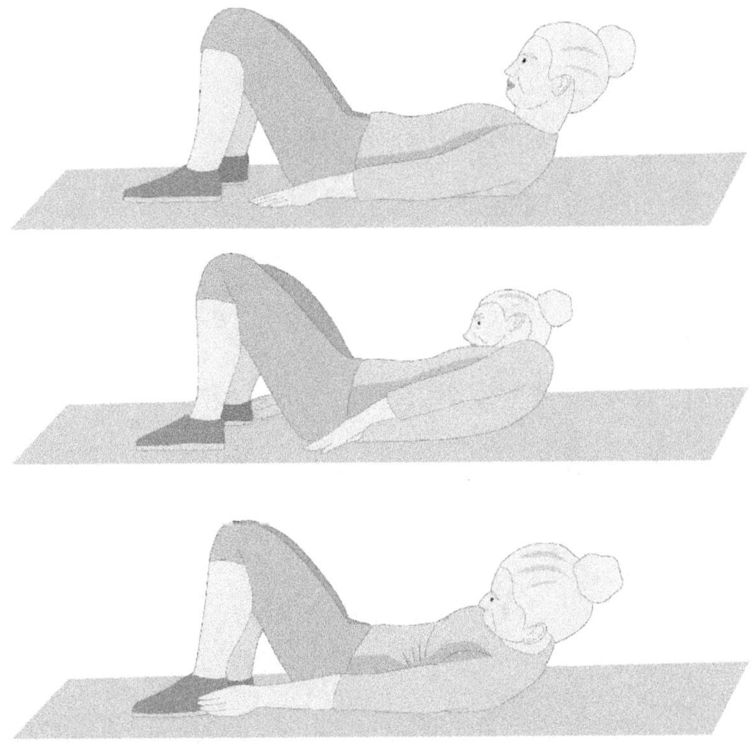

1. Lay down on the floor or a mat with your legs bent, feet flat on the floor
2. Place a rolled-up towel (or similar) underneath your lower back for support
3. Place each hand next to or behind the ears, but do not pull on your neck
   a. You can clasp them behind your head as well
4. Inhale and press your lower back into the towel
5. Exhaling slowly, bring your shoulders off the floor a bit and reach with your left arm down towards your left heel
6. Hold for 1-3 seconds
7. Return to start and reach for your right heel

Make is easier: Bring your feet closer to your hips, don't reach so far, leave your shoulders on the ground

Make it harder: Reach further to your toes, lift your shoulders high off of the ground, hold for up to 10 seconds.

Russian Twist

Muscles worked: rectus abdominis, transverse abdominis, hip flexors, latissimus dorsi, erector spinae

Be careful if: You have low-, mid-back, or hip issues

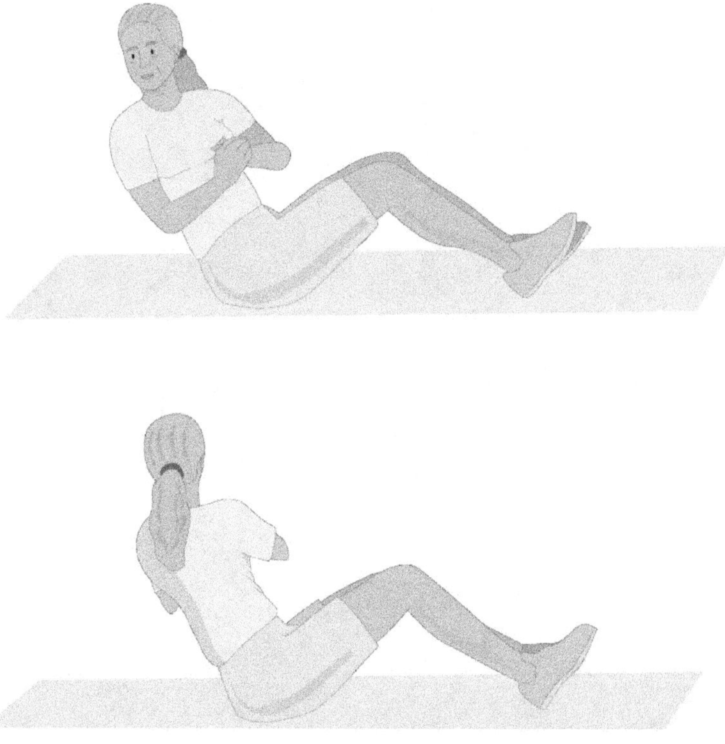

1. Sit on the floor or a mat with your legs bent, feet flat on the floor
2. Clasp hands in front of you or extend your arms out forward
3. Inhale and brace your core, lean back slightly so that your upper body is at a 45-degree angle to the floor
4. Exhaling slowly, twist your torso to your right as far as you can comfortably
5. Hold for 1-3 seconds and return to the center
6. Inhale and repeat the twist to your left

Make it easier: Straighten your legs out, lean back less

Make it harder: Sweep your arm back and behind you as you twist, lift your feet off of the ground, lean back more, sit on a folded towel or balance pad.

Floor Seated Knee Tuck

Muscles worked: rectus abdominis, transverse abdominis, hip flexors, erector spinae, psoas, external/internal obliques, quadriceps
Be careful if: you have hip or low-back issues

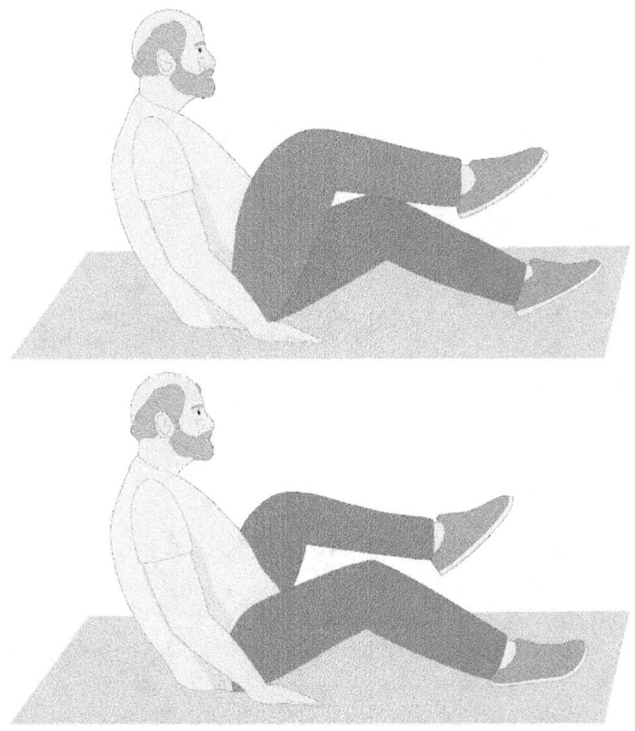

1. Sit up straight on the floor or a mat with your legs bent, feet flat on the floor
2. Clasp hands in front of you, extend your arms out forward, place your hands on your hips, or put them on the ground next to you
3. Sitting up tall, inhale and brace your core
4. Lift the left knee up towards the ceiling, exhaling slowly
5. Hold for 1-3 seconds
6. Return it back to the ground, switch legs and repeat

Make it easier: raise the heel instead of the whole foot off the ground, sit against a wall or place something behind your back to help stabilize your upper body

Make it harder: lift both knees at the same time, hold for up to 10 seconds, sit on a folded towel or balance pad.

Single Leg Lift

Muscles worked: rectus abdominis, transverse abdominis, psoas, external/internal oblique, hip flexors, quadriceps, hamstrings, erector spinae

Be careful if: You have low back or hip issues

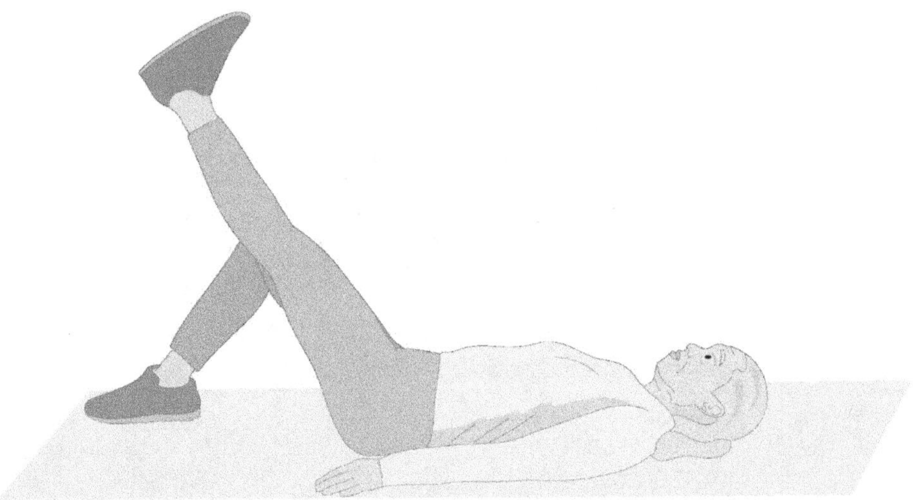

1) Lay on the floor or a mat with your knees up, feet flat on the floor
2) Place a rolled-up towel under your low back
3) Inhale, brace your core, press into the towel
   a) You can place your hands on your belly, to your side, or behind your head but don't pull on your neck
4) Exhaling, slowly raise one leg off of the floor to a count of 3-5
5) Lower it back to the ground slowly to a count of 3-5
6) Switch legs and repeat

Make it easier: Don't lift your leg as high, bend your knee more

Make it harder: Lift and lower for a count up to 10, bring your shoulders up off the ground, straighten your legs more, elevate your hips for a larger range of motion

Segmental Rotation (also Windshield Wiper)

Muscles worked: rectus abdominis, transverse abdominis, external/internal obliques, erector spinae, multifidus

Be careful if: You have low back, hip, knee, or ankle issues

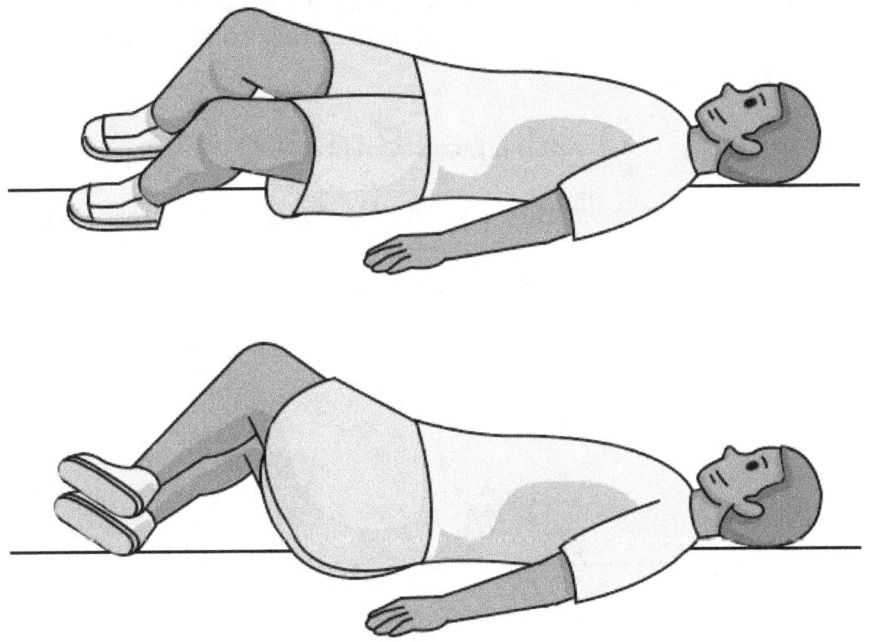

1. Lay on the floor or a mat with your knees up, feet flat on the floor
2. Place your hands, palm down, on the floor next to you or out to the side so your upper body forms a "T" shape.
3. Place a rolled-up towel (or similar) underneath your lower back for support
4. Inhale and press your lower back into the towel
5. Exhaling, slowly drop your knees to one side, only as far as is comfortable
6. Hold for 1-3 seconds, then bring the knees back to center and rotate them to the other side

Make it easier: Place pillows on either side of your knee for a higher surface, straighten your legs more, let one knee fall to the side instead of both

Make it harder: Bring your arms off of the floor, bring your feet off of the floor, straighten your legs more

PRONE (lying face down) EXERCISES

Prone, or face down, exercises work really well in combination with supine, or face up, exercises. Often, we focus only on core strength exercises that work the front of our body, however, focusing on the back of our body is really important, too. More so, we can train our body to resist forces from all directions and to make sure we aren't overtraining one area or group of muscles in our body. Prone exercises will help to train the spinal stabilizers to resist extension or too much frontward motion in the spine and help you to bring yourself back up from a bent forward or backward position

Quadruped Bird Dog

Muscles worked: erector spinae, multifidus, rectus abdominis, transverse abdominis, glutes

Be careful if: you have knee, hip, wrist, or shoulder issues

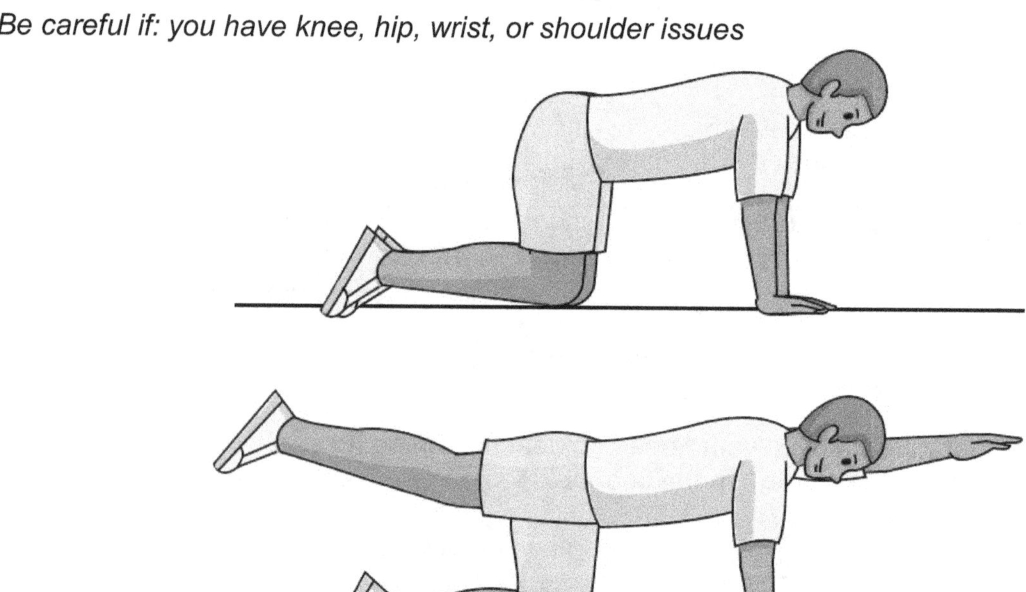

1) Come to all fours on the floor or a mat, shoulders stacked over hands, hips stacked over knees, keep your gaze a little out in front of your fingertips
2) Inhale and brace your core by performing a slight pelvic tilt (tuck your tailbone a bit) and draw your shoulder blades together
3) Lift your left knee and right hand off of the floor a few inches, exhaling slowly
    a) Try not to let your spine twist
4) Hold for 1-5 seconds
5) Slowly lower the hand and knee, switch sides and repeat
    a) Try to keep your hips from rocking as you make this transition

Make it easier: Raise the hand and knee individually, place your hands on an elevated surface, or hold for less time

Make it harder: Hold for up to 10 seconds, place an object on your back and balance it as you perform the move

Lying Hip Extension

Muscles worked: gluteus maximus/medius, hamstrings, hip flexors, erector spinae, transverse abdominis

Be careful if: you have hip or low-back issues

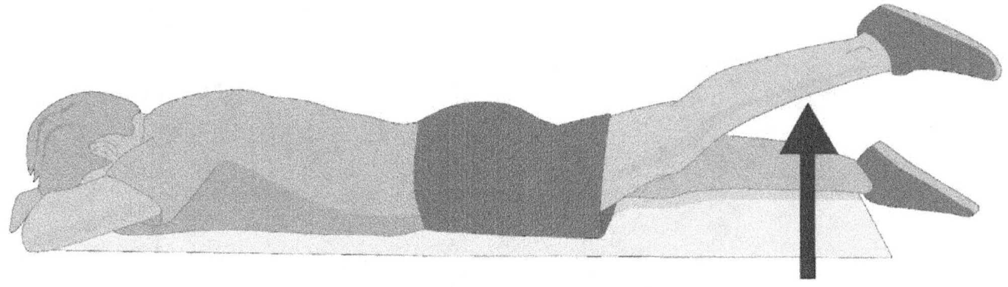

1. Lay face down on a floor or mat with your legs straight
2. Place your hands underneath your chin or your forehead
3. Inhale and brace your core
4. Lift your left leg up a few inches off of the ground from the hip, exhaling slowly
5. Hold for 1-3 seconds and return to the ground slowly
6. Inhale and repeat with the right leg

Make it easier: If you cannot get your leg off of the floor, simply squeeze the glute of the left leg, then the right, bend the knee of the leg you are lifting off of the ground

Make it harder: Hold for up to 10 seconds, pulse the leg up and down, elevate the hips to increase the range of motion

Donkey Kick

Muscles worked: gluteus maximus, hamstrings, rectus abdominis, external/internal obliques, transverse abdominis, erector spinae

Be careful if: You have knee, hip, or low-back issues

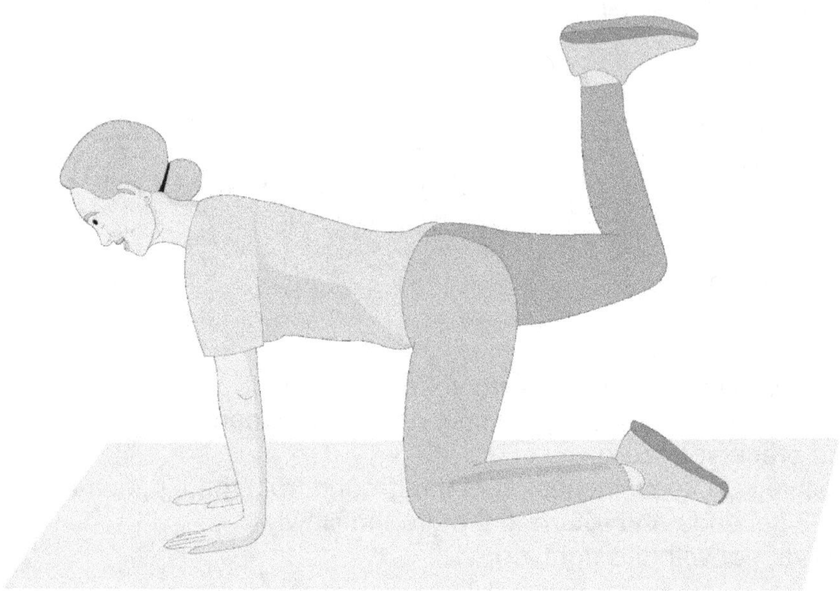

1. Come to all fours on the floor or a mat, shoulders stacked over hands, hips stacked over knees, keep your gaze a little out in front of your fingertips
2. Inhale and brace your core by performing a slight pelvic tilt (tuck your tailbone a bit) and draw your shoulder blades together
3. Leading with your heel, lift your left leg (knee stays bent) straight up towards the ceiling, exhaling slowly
4. Hold for 1-3 seconds
5. Return to start and repeat with opposite leg

Make it easier: Lift the leg less

Make it harder: Hold for up to 10 seconds, wear an ankle weight, pulse the lifted leg

Alternating Superman

Muscles worked: erector spinae, rectus abdominis, transverse abdominis, hamstrings, gluteus maximus, trapezius, deltoids (shoulders)

Be careful if: you have hip, low-, or mid-back issues

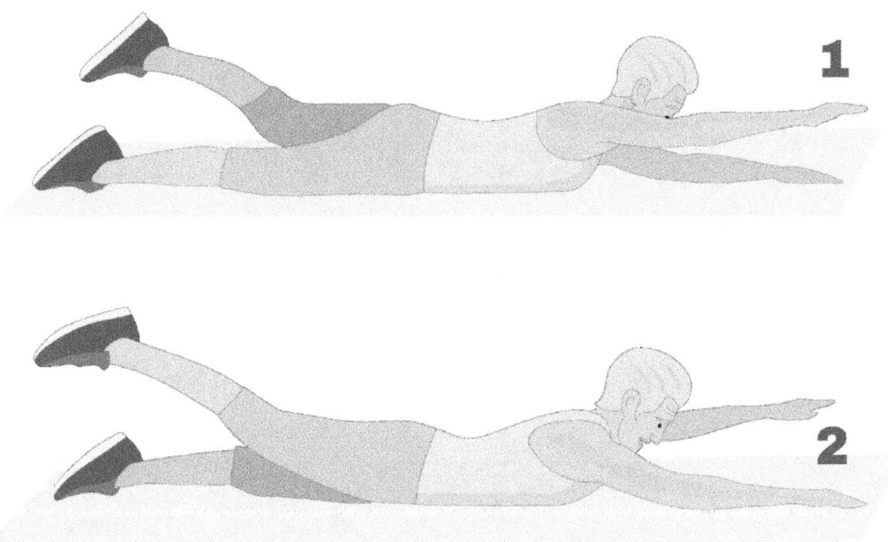

1. Lay face down on a floor or mat with your legs straight
2. Place your arms straight out in front of you or bend your arm at the elbow to create a goal-post shape with your arms
3. Inhale and brace your core
4. Lift your left leg (from the hip) and right arm (from the shoulder) up a few inches off of the ground, exhaling slowly. Note: You're always lifting opposing limbs.
5. Hold for 1-3 seconds and return to the ground slowly
6. Inhale and repeat with the right leg and left arm

Make is easier: Raise arms and legs separately

Make it harder: Raise both arms and legs at the same time, hold for up to 10 seconds, and elevate your hips for a larger range of motion.

As with most anything in life, variety is a great idea! You know your body better than anyone, so choose with your ability and goal in mind and err on the side of caution. It's easier to increase the challenge than to have challenged yourself too much. If you potentially injure yourself or you are way too sore, then you have to take a lot of time to recover which puts a huge damper on your progress. It's also a good idea to choose exercises from each of these categories; however, they may not all work for you. Try them all out and see what works best for you. Oftentimes, the ones that are the most challenging tend to be the ones we need to work on the most! However, that isn't always the case.

The variations listed are by no means the only way to change these exercises to make them easier or more challenging. Keep in mind when you attempt each exercise, take it slow and stay mindful about how you feel before, during, and after. Additionally, if you attempt to make an exercise easier or more challenging, only change one thing at a time. If you make too many modifications all at once, you can't be sure which modification worked better or worse. Bear in mind noticeable changes take time, so be patient with yourself, give yourself some grace, and remain consistent!

CHAPTER 9 - Chair Core Exercises

As we age, balance and stability can decline. This can make working out even more challenging. The good news is that there's an alternative to traditional floor or mat-based core exercises that can be performed from a chair while still retaining all of the benefits! Using the chair to increase stability and balance can boost confidence during each exercise, making movement safer and more effective. Remember, your body will preferentially use energy to ensure you don't fall down. But this extra energy expenditure means less energy available for each exercise. By removing the unstable piece of the puzzle and planting yourself in a chair, you can more easily focus on the tasks at hand.

Ideally, you will want a stable, sturdy chair without arms - a wooden dining room chair is perfect! Couches and loveseats tend not to work as well because they're too soft to offer support during movement, though if that's your only option, then use it.

If you already perform a strength routine, and do not focus on core work specifically, then a rule of thumb is to add two to three, core specific routines per week. Bear in mind, how often you strength train as extra core specific work can fatigue larger muscle groups and that can affect your other training negatively. If you are unsure, add in one core specific routine per week and add one or two from there.

Perform one to three sets of each exercise, aiming for 12-15 quality repetitions of each. You can break these repetitions up if you need to, or make the repetition range a goal.

Seated Knee Tuck

Muscles worked: rectus abdominis, transverse abdominis, hip flexors, erector spinae, psoas, external/internal obliques, quadriceps

Be careful if: you have hip or low-back issues

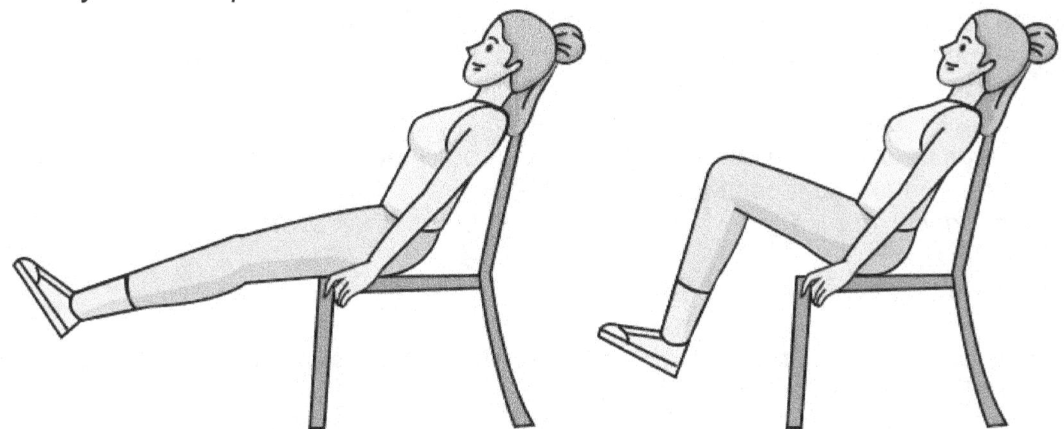

1. Sit in the middle of the chair, feet flat on the floor
2. Clasp hands in front of you, extend your arms out forward, place your hands on your hips, or hold on to the edge of the chair for balance
3. Sitting up tall, inhale and brace your core (pelvic tilt)
4. Lift both knees towards your chest and hold for 1-3 seconds, exhaling slowly

5. Return your feet to the ground and repeat

Make it easier: don't bring the knees so high, perform with one leg at a time, lean back further

Make it harder: hold for up to 10 seconds, do not put your feet back on the ground in between tucks

Seated Scissor Kick

Muscles worked: rectus abdominis, transverse abdominis, hip flexors, erector spinae, psoas, external/internal obliques, quadriceps, gluteus maximus/medius

Be careful if: you have hip or low-back issues

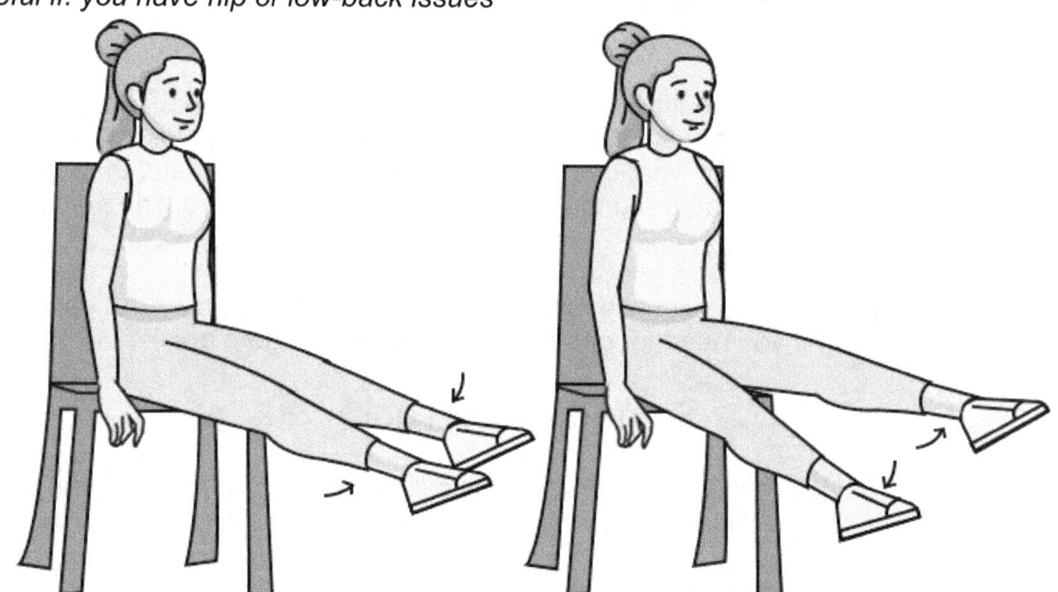

1) Sit in the middle of the chair, legs extended out in front of you
2) Clasp hands in front of you, extend your arms out forward, place your hands on your hips, or hold on to the edge of the chair for balance
3) Sitting up tall, inhale and brace your core (pelvic tilt)
4) Lift both legs up off of the floor and spread them out wide, slowly, then bring them back towards the center and cross them a bit, exhaling
   a) *Variation: lift your left leg while your right leg drops, then switch, right leg up, left leg down, repeat*
5) Return them to the floor and repeat

Make it easier: don't lift the legs so high, bend the knees a bit, perform with one leg at a time or hold one leg still while you move the other one

Make it harder: move more slowly, don't put your legs down between repetitions, hold in the outer and inner positions for up to 10 seconds

Seated Twist (add in palm press)

Muscles worked: rectus abdominis, transverse abdominis, hip flexors, latissimus dorsi, erector spinae, pectoralis major (chest)

Be careful if: you have low- or mid-back issues

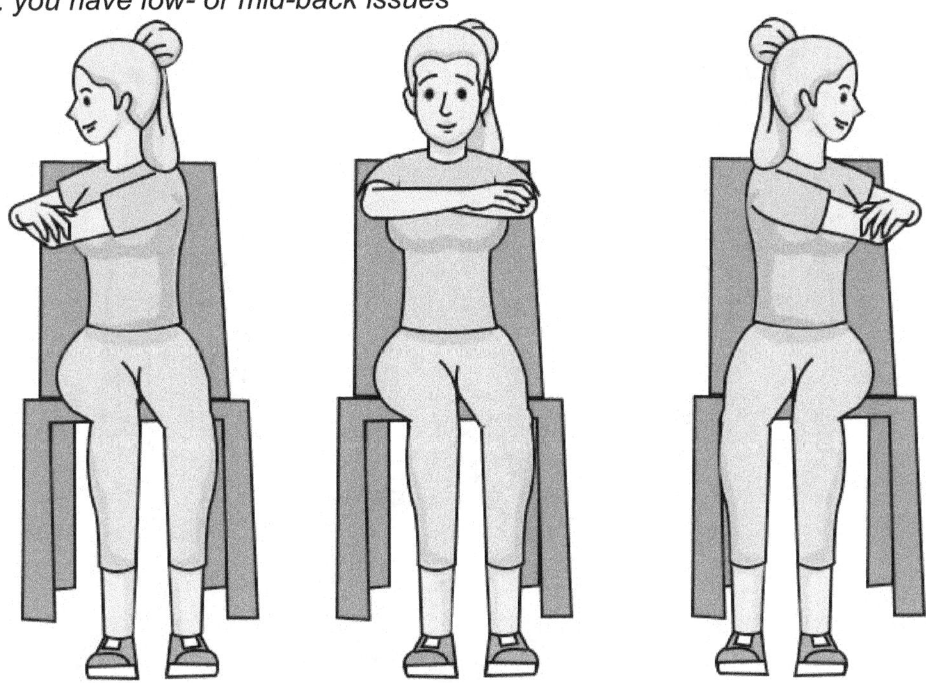

1. Sit in the middle of the chair, feet flat on the floor
2. Place your hands on your hips, fold them in front of you, or clasp them in front of you
3. Sitting up tall, inhale and brace your core (pelvic tilt)
4. Slowly twist to the right and hold for 1-3 seconds, exhaling
5. Inhale as you come back to center and twist the opposite direction

Make it easier: brace a little less, don't twist as much

Make it harder: press your palms together further engaging your core, hold for up to 10 seconds, lift one or both feet off the floor

Clock Bends

Muscles worked: Muscles worked: external/internal obliques, transverse abdominals, rectus abdominis, quadratus lumborum

Be careful if: you have low-back issues

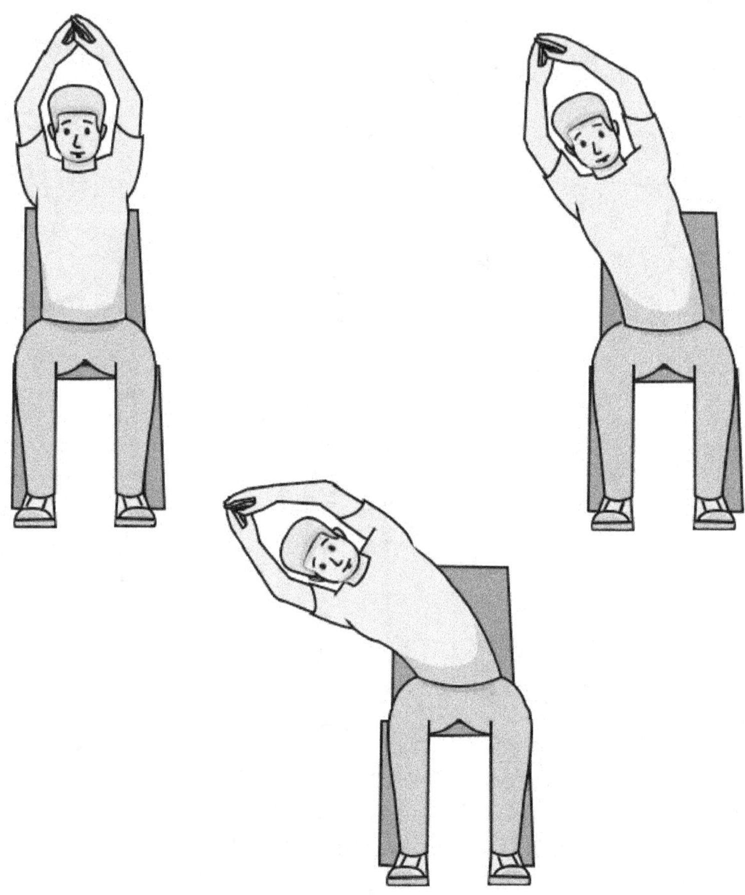

1) Sit in the middle of the chair, feet flat on the floor
2) Raise your arms up overhead and place your palms together
3) Sitting up tall, inhale and brace your core (pelvic tilt)
4) Imagine you are in the center of a clock, where noon is behind you
5) Lean slowly towards each "time" on the clock, exhaling slowly
   a) For example; lean forward towards 6 o'clock, come back to center, then lean towards 5 o'clock and so forth.

Make it easier: Don't sway as far, bring your arms down, or hold onto the edge of the chair as you sway

Make it harder: Hold weight in your hands, bring the leg opposite the side you are leaning off the ground

Elbow to Knee

Muscles worked: external/internal obliques, rectus abdominis, transverse abdominis, hip flexors, quadriceps, hamstrings

Be careful if: you have hip, low-, or mid-back issues

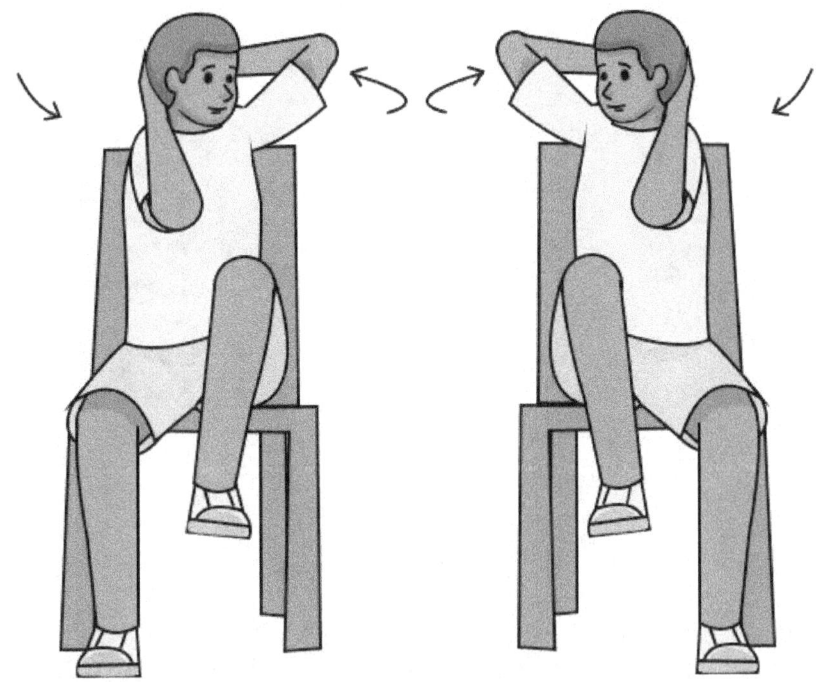

1) Sit in the middle of the chair, feet flat on the floor
2) Place each hand next to or behind the ears, but do not pull on your neck
   a) You can clasp them behind your head as well
3) Sitting up tall, inhale and brace your core (pelvic tilt)
4) Slowly pull your left knee towards your head and reach your right elbow towards the knee, exhaling slowly
   a) The elbow and knee do not have to touch, get them as close together as you can without pain or discomfort
5) Hold for 1-3 seconds
6) Return to start, switch legs and arms and repeat

Make it easier: reach with your hand instead of your elbow, don't lift the knee as high.

Make it harder: touch the elbow to the knee.

Seated Forward Fold

Muscles worked: erector spinae, rectus abdominis, transverse abdominis, gluteus maximus, hip flexors

Be careful if: you have low-back issues

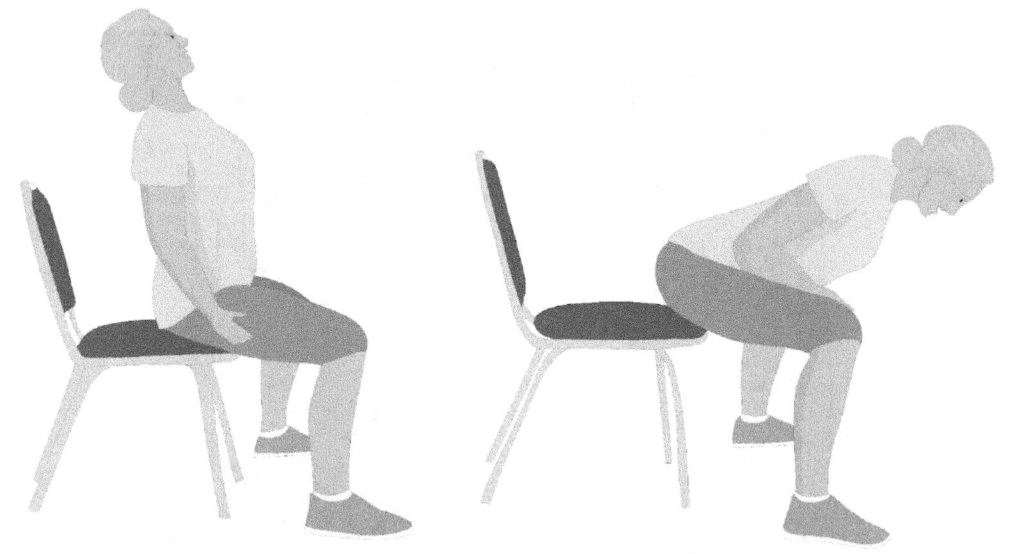

1) Sit in the middle of the chair, feet flat on the floor, legs wider than the chair legs
2) Place your hands on your hips or on your legs
3) Sitting up tall, inhale and brace your core (pelvic tilt)
4) Slowly bend at the hip, moving your upper body as one single unit, exhaling slowly
    a) Only go as far forward as you feel comfortable
5) Pause for 1-3 seconds, squeeze your glutes, and return to an upright position

Make it easier: use your hands to brace yourself as you lower, don't fold as far forward

Make it harder: put your arms above your head, hold a small weight in front of your chest, bend further, hold for up to 10 seconds

Knee Lift

Muscles worked: rectus abdominis, transverse abdominis, hip flexors, erector spinae, psoas, external/internal obliques, quadriceps

Be careful if: you have hip or low-back issues

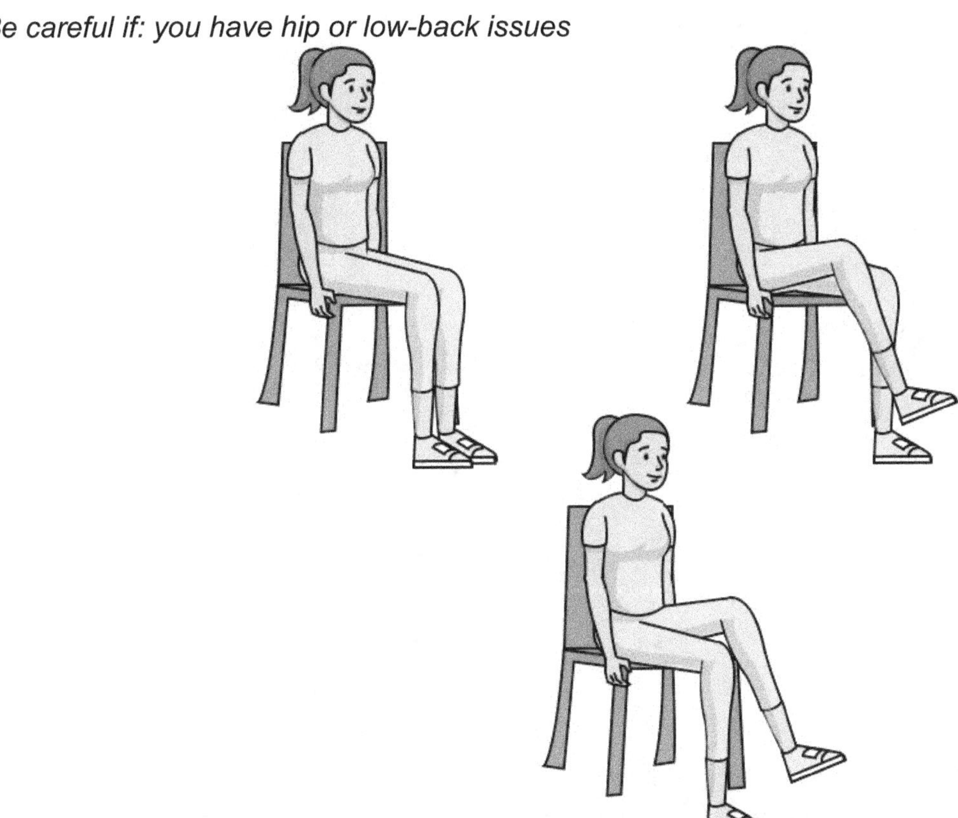

1. Sit in the middle of the chair, feet flat on the floor
2. Clasp your hands in front of you, extend your arms out forward, place your hands on your hips, or hold on to the edge of the chair for balance
3. Sitting up tall, inhale and brace your core (pelvic tilt)
4. Lift your left knee up towards the ceiling, exhaling slowly
5. Hold for 1-3 seconds
6. Return it back to the ground, switch legs and repeat

Make it easier: raise the heel instead of the whole foot off the ground, sit against a wall or place something behind your back to help stabilize your upper body

Make it harder: lift both knees at the same time, hold for up to 10 seconds, sit on a folded towel or balance pad

Leg Lift

Muscles worked: rectus abdominis, transverse abdominis, psoas, external/internal oblique, hip flexors, quadriceps, hamstrings, erector spinae

Be careful if: you have low back or hip issues

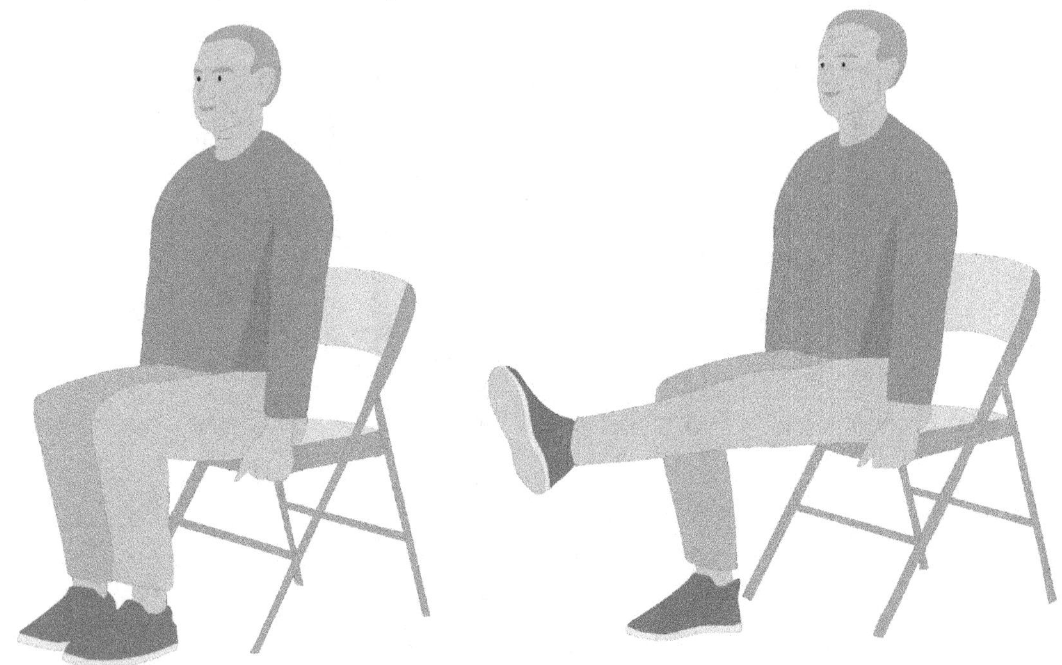

1. Sit in the middle of the chair, right foot flat on the floor, left leg extended
2. Clasp hands in front of you, extend your arms out forward, place your hands on your hips, or hold on to the edge of the chair for balance
3. Sitting up tall, inhale and brace your core (pelvic tilt)
4. Lift your left leg up towards the ceiling, exhaling slowly
5. Hold for 1-3 seconds
6. Return it back to the ground, switch legs and repeat

Make it easier: don't lift the leg as high, bend the knee a bit

Make it harder: hold the leg for up to 10 seconds, lift the leg higher

Knee Bending (also Knee Tuck)

Muscles worked: rectus abdominis, transverse abdominis, hip flexors, erector spinae, psoas, external/internal obliques, quadriceps

Be careful if: you have hip or low-back issues

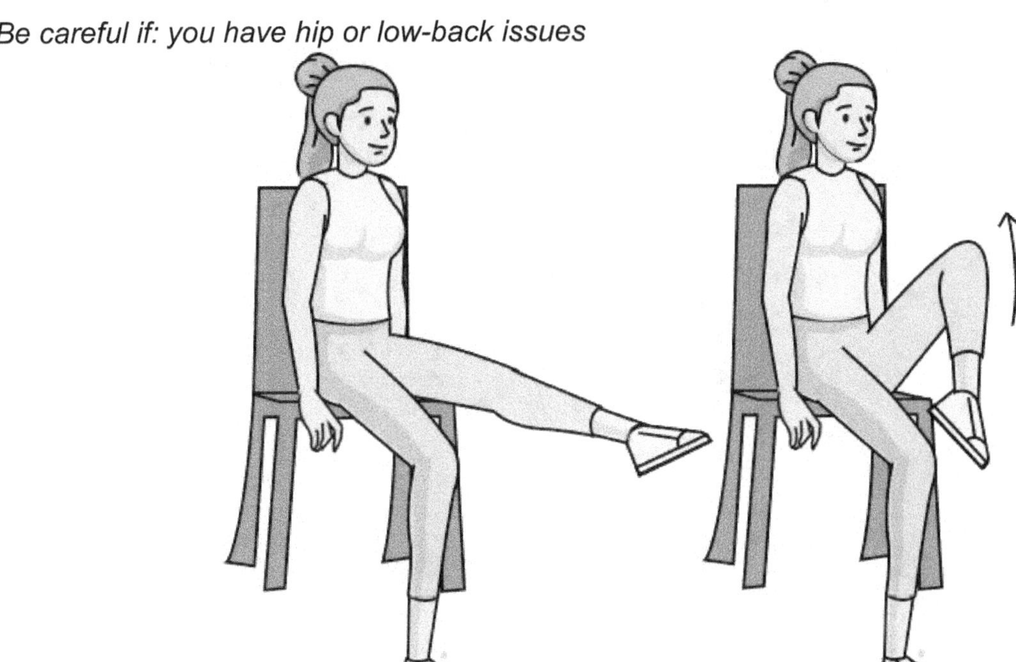

1. Sit in the middle of the chair, left foot flat on the floor, right leg extended
2. Clasp hands in front of you, extend your arms out forward, place your hands on your hips, or hold on to the edge of the chair for balance
3. Sitting up tall, inhale and brace your core (pelvic tilt)
4. Lift your left leg up until parallel with the floor then bend the knee to bring it towards your chest, exhaling slowly
5. Hold for 1-3 seconds
6. Return it back to the ground, switch legs and repeat

Make it easier: don't lift the leg so high, bend the knee more at the start, elevate the working leg so you begin with it higher off the ground

Make it harder: elevate both legs, hold for up to 10 second

Elevated Chair Plank

Muscles worked: rectus abdominis, external/internal obliques, transverse abdominis, erector spinae, trapezius, latissimus dorsi, pectorals (chest muscles), serratus anterior, deltoids, biceps, triceps, glutes, hamstrings, and quads

Be careful if: you have shoulder, elbow, neck, low-, mid-, low-back, knee or hip issues

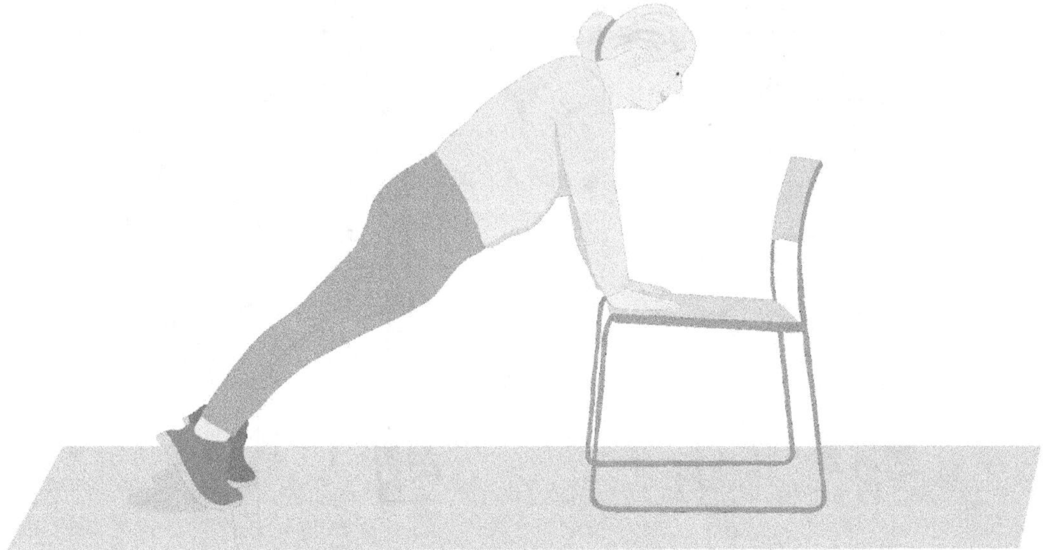

1) Place a chair against a wall so it doesn't slide
2) Place your hands on the seat of the chair, thumbs on top or below the seat
3) Your elbows should be stacked underneath your shoulders
4) Inhale, contract your core and glutes (perform a pelvic tilt) and extend both legs out behind you so they are straight
5) Maintain a neutral spine and neck by looking a foot in front of you and keep your tailbone tucked so your hips do not sag or poke up too far
   a) It's called a plank because you should be straight as a board from the back of your head to your toes
6) Hold this position for as long as you can maintain proper form, up to 30 seconds

Make it easier: Bring one or both feet closer to the chair, turn the chair around and use the back of the chair

Make it harder: Lift one foot off the ground, lift one hand off the chair seat, rock your hips gently from side to side

Seated Bicycle

Muscles worked: rectus abdominis, transverse abdominis, hip flexors, erector spinae, psoas, external/internal obliques, quadriceps, hamstrings, gluteus maximus/medius

Be careful if: you have hip or low-back issues

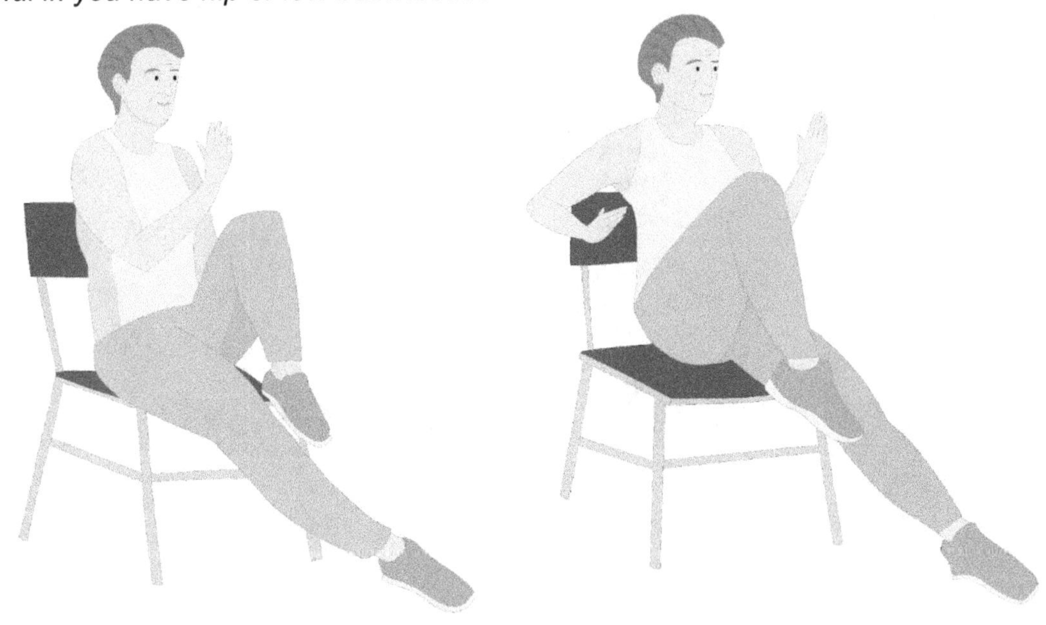

1. Sit in the middle of the chair, feet flat on the floor
2. Clasp your hands in front of you, extend your arms out forward, place your hands on your hips, or hold on to the edge of the chair for balance
3. Sitting up tall, inhale and brace your core (pelvic tilt)
4. Lift both knees up towards the ceiling a bit and begin to "pedal" your feet in the air, exhaling, slowly for 1-3 revolutions per leg
5. Lower them to the ground and repeat

Make it easier: pedal with one leg at a time, don't lift your legs as high, lean back into the chair further

Make it harder: sit up straighter, "pedal" more slowly

Seated Pelvic Tilt (Anterior & Posterior)

Muscles worked: quadriceps, erector spinae, multifidus, quadratus lumborum, external/internal oblique, psoas (anterior), hamstring, quadriceps, gluteus maximus/medius, rectus abdominis, external/internal oblique (posterior)

Be careful if: you have low back issues

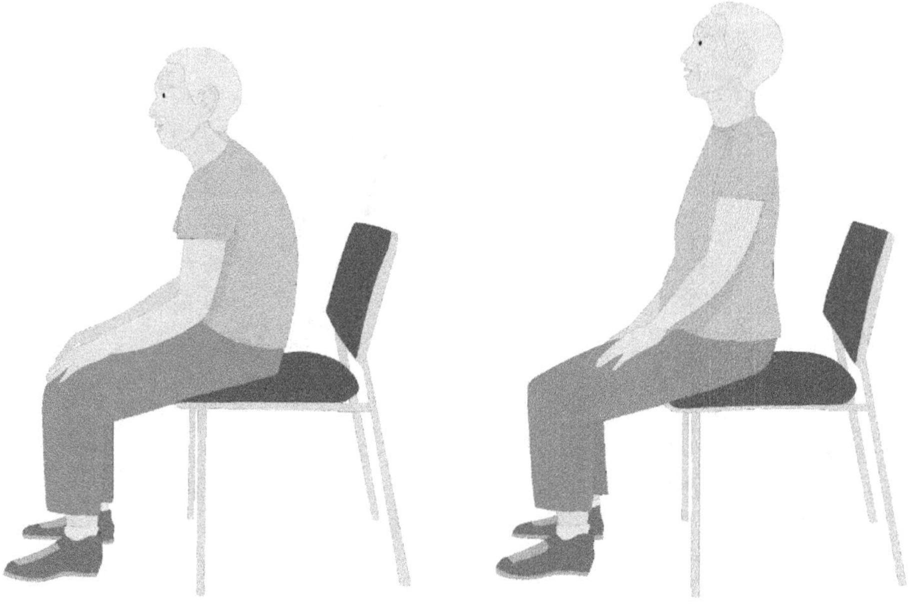

1. Sit in the middle of the chair, feet flat on the floor
2. Place your hands on your hips

(Posterior Pelvic Tilt)
1. Inhale and slowly rock the top of your hips back and tuck your tailbone under, you'll feel yourself curling forwards a bit
2. Hold for 1-3 seconds, exhaling slowly

(Anterior Pelvic Tilt)
1. Inhale and begin to reverse this motion
2. Exhale slowly and begin to slowly stick your tailbone "out" or behind you
3. Hold for 1-3 seconds

Make it easier: sit on a folded-up towel for more feedback as to how your pelvis is moving

Make it harder: pick your feet up off of the floor

Seated Russian Twist

Muscles worked: rectus abdominis, transverse abdominis, hip flexors, latissimus dorsi, erector spinae

Be careful if: you have low-, mid-back, or hip issues

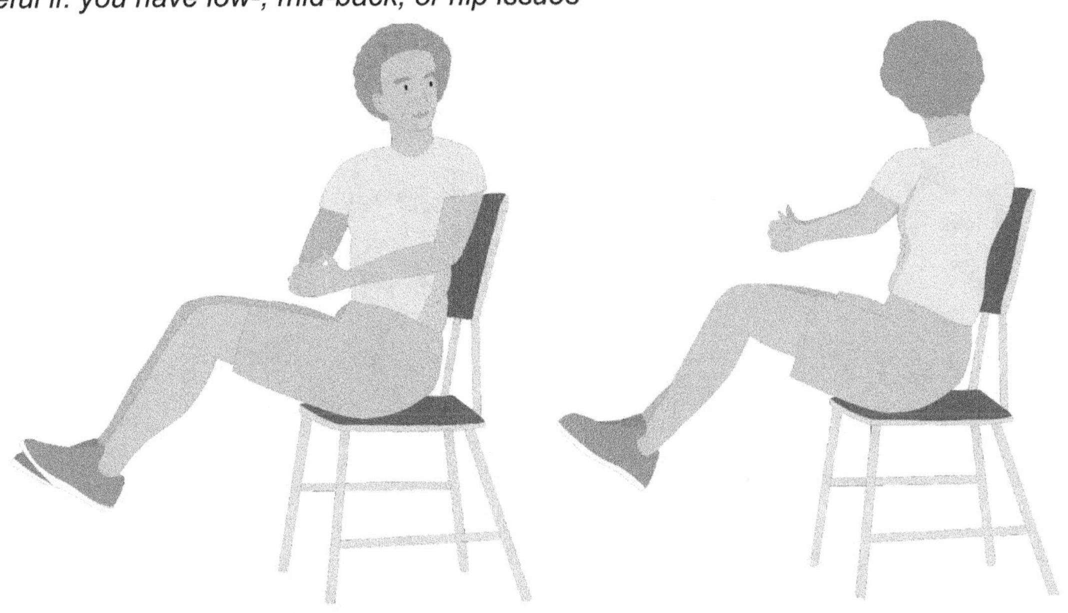

1. Sit in the middle of the chair, legs extended a bit
2. Clasp hands in front of you, extend your arms out forward, place your hands on your hips, or hold on to the edge of the chair for balance
3. Sitting up tall, inhale, brace your core (pelvic tilt) and lean back slightly
4. Exhaling slowly, twist to your right as far as you comfortably can
5. Hold for 1-3 seconds and return to the center
6. Inhale and repeat the twist to your left

Make it easier: Bend your knees more, lean back less

Make it harder: Sweep your arm back and behind you as you twist, lift your feet off of the ground, lean back more, sit on a folded towel or balance pad

Seated Single Leg Abdominal Press (instead of Knee to Knee)

Muscles worked: transverse abdominis, external/internal obliques, quadriceps, hip flexors

Be careful if: you have low back, knee, or shoulder issues

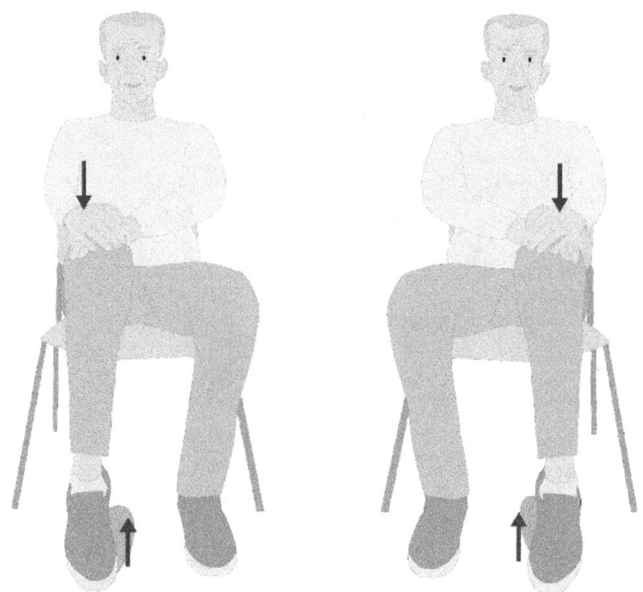

1. Sit in the middle of the chair, feet flat on the floor
2. Place your hands on your legs
3. Sitting up tall, inhale and brace your core (pelvic tilt)
4. Press your right knee into your right hand and hold for 1-3 seconds, exhaling slowly
5. Release and switch to your left knee and hand

Make it easier: don't press so hard, press down with your hand only

Make it harder: press harder, hold up to 10 seconds, bring both feet off of the ground

Metronome

Muscles worked: external/internal obliques, transverse abdominals, rectus abdominis, quadratus lumborum
Be careful if: you have low-back issues

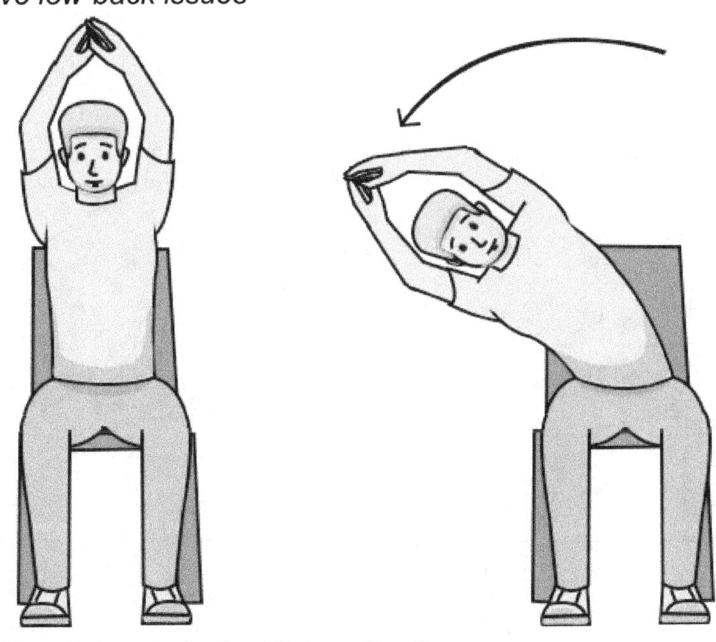

1. Sit in the middle of the chair, feet flat on the floor
2. Raise your arms up overhead and place your palms together
3. Sitting up tall, inhale and brace your core (pelvic tilt)
4. Lean slowly to your left as far as you comfortably can, exhaling slowly
5. When you can't lean to the left anymore, pause briefly and begin to sway to the other side (like a metronome)

Make it easier: Don't sway as far, bring your arms down, or hold onto the edge of the chair as you sway

Make it harder: Hold weight in your hands, bring the leg opposite the side you are leaning off the ground

Chair Glute Bridge

Muscles worked: transverse abdominis, gluteus maximus, erector spinae, hamstrings

Be careful if: you have low-back issues

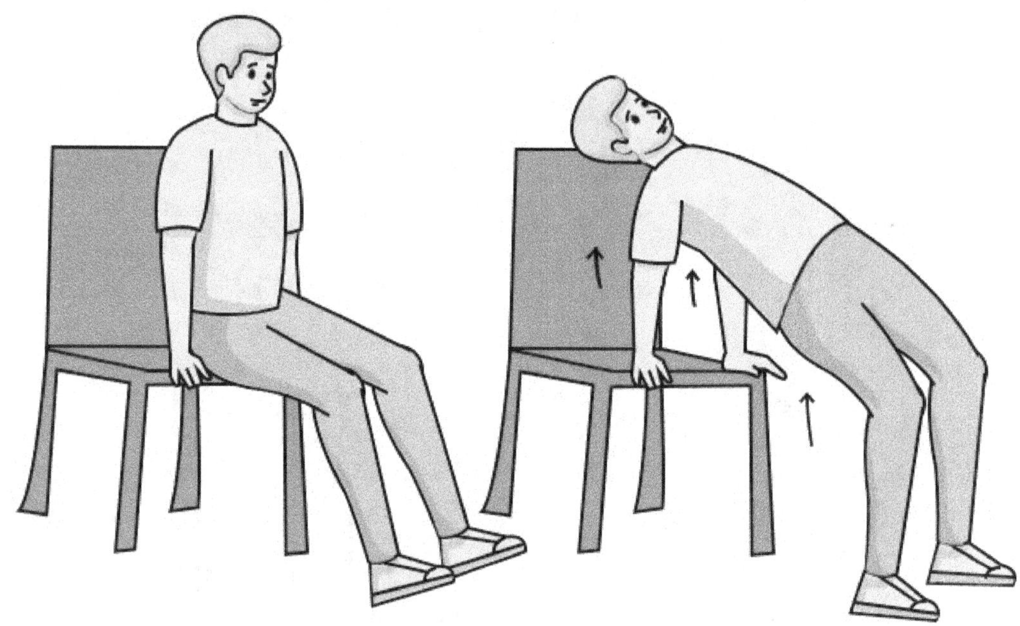

1. Sit in the middle of the chair, feet flat on the floor
2. Place the heels of your hands on to the side edge of the chair
3. Sitting up tall, inhale and brace your core (pelvic tilt)
4. Squeeze your glutes (butt) and bring your hips into the air, hold for 1-3 seconds, exhaling slowly
5. Return to the chair and repeat

Make it easier: Don't lift the hips as high

Make it harder: Hold for up to 10 seconds, pick one (or both) leg up off of the ground

Side Bends

Muscles worked: external/internal obliques, transverse abdominals, rectus abdominis, quadratus lumborum

Be careful if: you have low-back issues

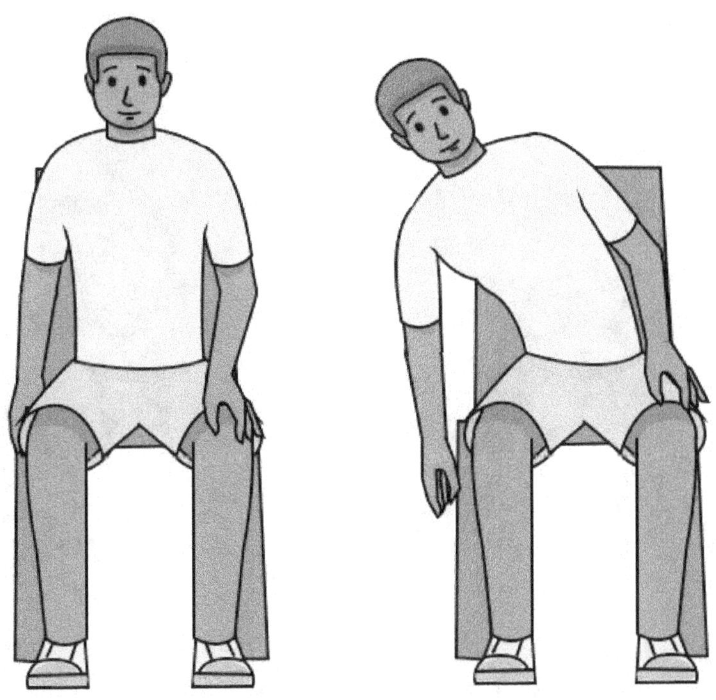

1. Sit in the middle of the chair, feet flat on the floor
2. Clasp your hands in front of you, place your hands on your hips, hold on to the side edge of the chair, or let your arms hang to your sides
3. Sitting up tall, inhale and brace your core (pelvic tilt)
4. Lean slowly to your left as far as you comfortably can, exhaling slowly
5. Hold for 1-3 seconds
6. Return back upright, switch sides and repeat

Make it easier: Don't lean as far, hold on to the opposite edge of the chair you are leaning.

Make it harder: Hold for up to 10 seconds, put arms up in the air or out to your sides, hold weight in your hand

Heel to Toe Tap

Muscles worked: quadratus lumborum, transverse abdominis, psoas, hip flexors

Be careful if: you have hip or knee issues

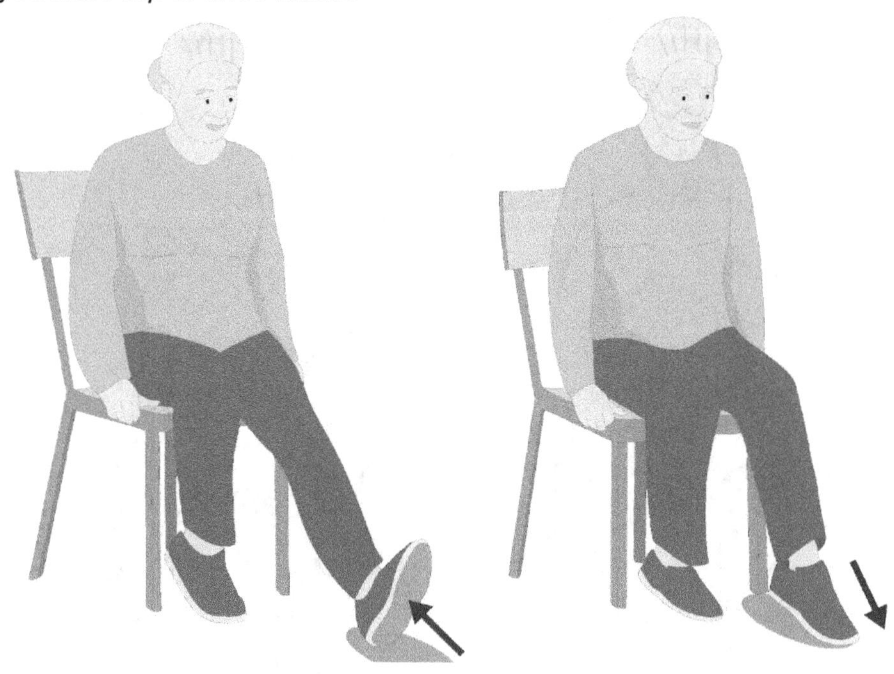

1. Sit in the middle of the chair, feet flat on the floor
2. Place your hands on your legs
3. Sitting up tall, inhale and brace your core (pelvic tilt)
4. Extend your right leg and tap your heel on the ground, bend your knee and tap your toe underneath you, exhaling slowly
5. Switch legs and repeat

Make it easier: place a towel under your foot so it glides, perform the heel and toe taps separately

Make it harder: bring the knee up higher during the hell to toe transition, keep the opposite leg off of the ground

Seated Side Crunch

Muscles worked: external/internal oblique, hip flexors

Be careful if: you have low-back or hip issues

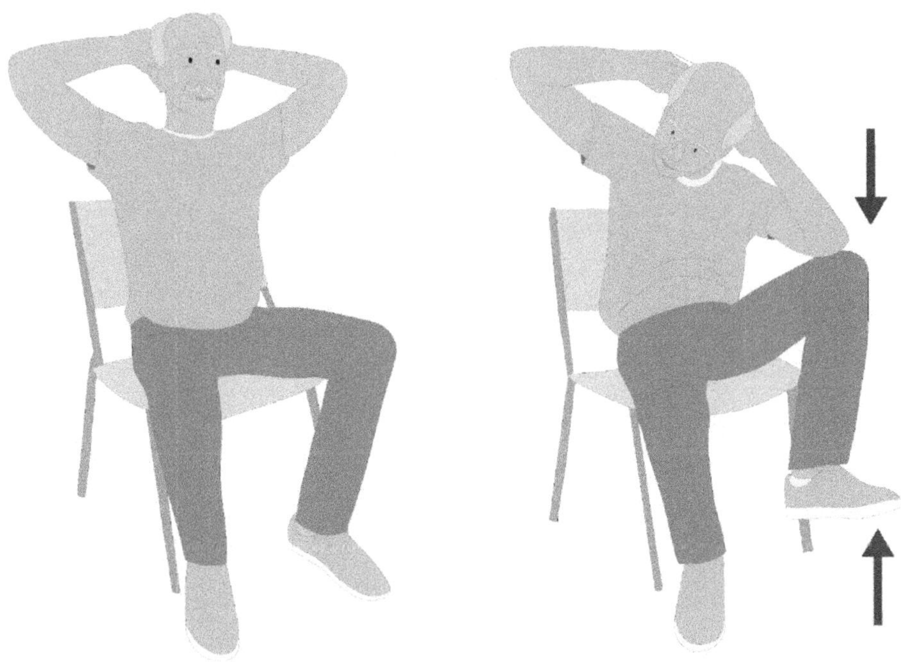

1) Sit in the middle of the chair, legs wider than the chair legs, feet flat on the floor
2) Place each hand next to or behind the ears but do not pull on your neck
   a) You can clasp them behind your head as well
3) Sitting up tall, inhale and brace your core (pelvic tilt)
4) Bend sideways to your left a bit and lift your left knee towards your left elbow, hold for 1-3 seconds, exhaling slowly
5) Return your foot to the ground and repeat with the right leg

Make it easier: Don't lift the knee as high, don't bend sideways as far, hold on to the opposite edge of the chair for stability

Make it harder: Hold for up to 10 seconds, bring the elbow and knee closer together

Do not be fooled by the fact that these are chair exercises. They can be very challenging if you choose to make them so. That being said, it is nearly always best to choose a standing or floor option when you can to maximize the benefit of each exercise. Chair, or seated, exercises are most often options for safety reasons, not necessarily because someone isn't capable of other types of exercise. Again, do not be fooled into thinking these exercises are inherently easy. Like anything in life, we often get back what we put in. If you are keeping your safety in mind by choosing seated core exercises, then you have set yourself up safely to challenge yourself and be all the better for it. However, if you need the seated exercises because a floor exercise or other variation is too difficult then kudos to you for choosing wisely. We all begin somewhere different on our strength journey, and where we feel the safest and most confident is typically the best starting point. You know your body better than anyone, so use this knowledge about yourself to your advantage. If you are unsure, seated core exercises are a great starting point on your fitness journey.

Chapter 10 - Standing Core Exercises

Standing exercises can be a great middle ground between floor and chair exercises and are often chosen due to their wider range of difficulty. With exercise in general, you get out of it what you put into it. Standing core exercises are considered more functional than other forms because most of the activities we perform on a daily basis take from a standing position. If this is how we execute daily tasks and move around, why not train that way? If you choose to perform standing core exercises, you will be giving your body useful feedback about how it moves while in an upright position. It also gives those who do not feel comfortable or safe getting down to the ground another option!

If you already perform a strength routine and do not focus on core work specifically, then a rule of thumb is to add two to three core-specific routines per week. Bear in mind how often you strength train, as extra core-specific work can fatigue larger muscle groups. If you don't have enough time to recover between workouts, this extra stress on your core muscles could negatively affect your other training. Start with one core routine per week and increase from there if things go well.

Perform one to three sets of each exercise you choose. Aim for 12-15 quality repetitions of each. You can break these repetitions up if you need to, or make the repetition range a goal.

Standing Bird Dog

Muscles worked: Rectus abdominis, transverse abdominis, erector spinae, latissimus dorsi, hip flexors, hamstrings, gluteus maximus
Be careful if: You have hip, back, or shoulder issues

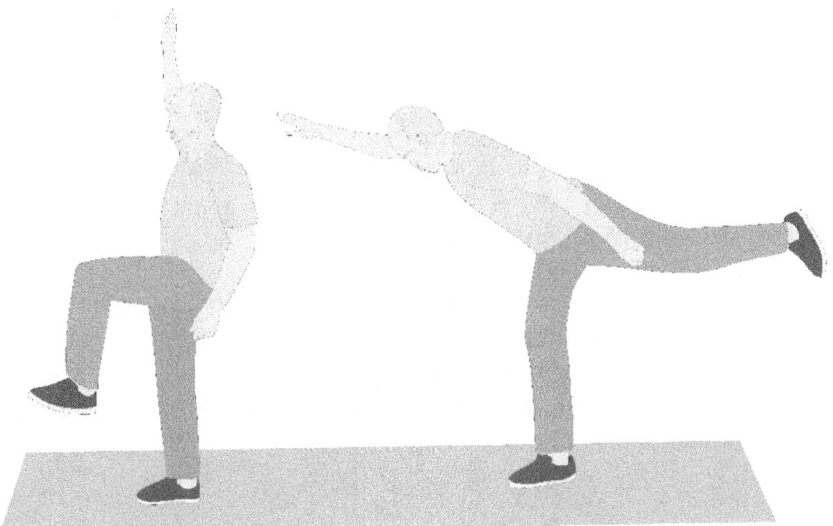

1) Stand upright and tall, feet about shoulder-width apart
   a) Stand near a wall for stability
2) Inhale and brace your core (pelvic tilt)

3) Lift your left knee close to hip height and raise your right arm overhead, exhaling slowly
4) Hinge at the hip, going as far as parallel with the ground
5) Hold for 1-3 seconds
6) Return back to start, switch sides, and repeat

Make it easier: Do not bend forward as much or at all, hold on to the back of a chair or counter top

Make it harder: hold for up to 10 seconds, draw the opposite knee and elbow together slowly.

Standing Crunch

Works: Rectus abdominis, erector spinae, transverse abdominis, external/internal obliques

Be careful if: You have neck, mid-, or lower back issues

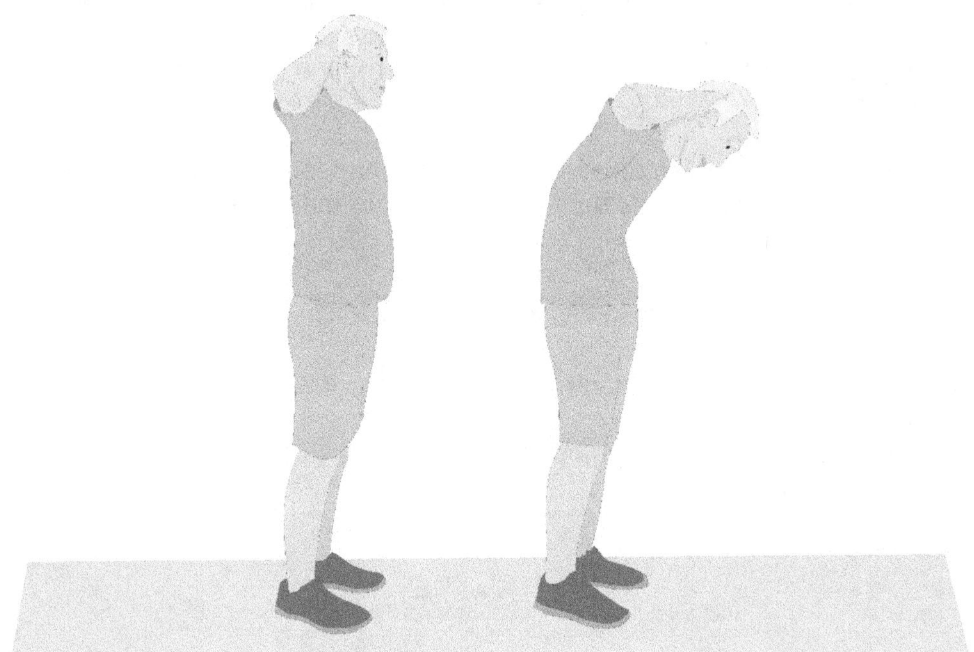

1) Stand upright and tall, feet about shoulder-width apart
    a) Stand against a wall for stability
2) Place your hands behind your ears, behind your head, or on your hips
    a) Do not pull on your head or neck
3) Inhale and brace your core (posterior pelvic tilt)
4) Curl your upper body down as far as you can comfortably go, exhaling slowly
    a) Keep your hips stationary
5) Hold for 1-3 seconds
6) Return back to start and repeat

Make it easier: Do not curl down as far, place a rolled-up towel behind your back and against a wall to keep your lower body stationary

Make it harder: Hold for up to 10 seconds, curl further forward, hold weight in front of chest

Windmill

Muscles worked: Deltoids, rhomboids, trapezius, rectus abdominis, external/internal obliques, erector spinae, pelvic floor, diaphragm, gluteus maximus, hamstring

Be careful if: You have shoulder, low-back, or hip issues

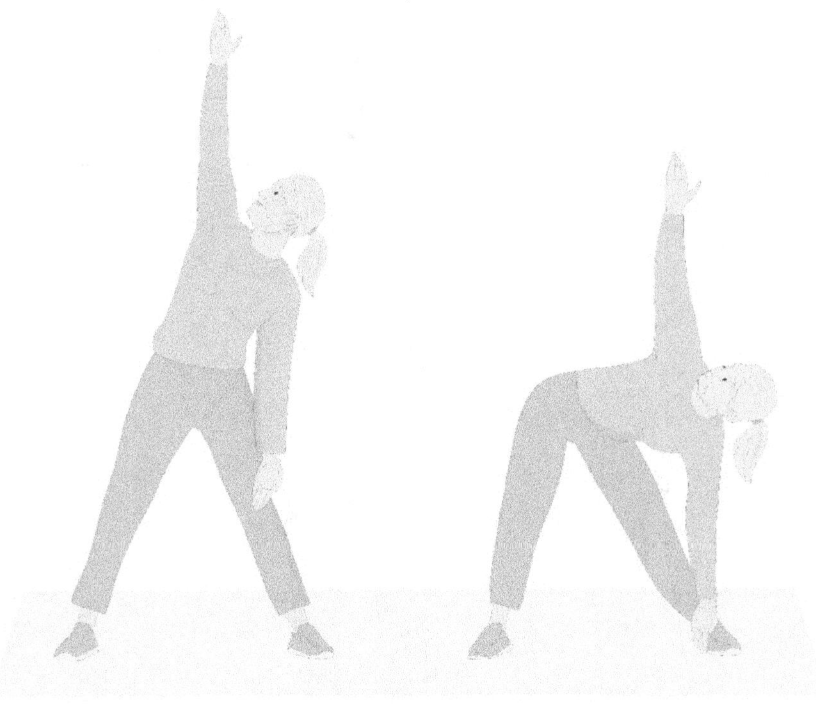

1) Stand up nice and tall with your feet wider than your shoulders, left foot angled outward, around a 45° angle
2) Raise your right arm straight up and overhead, and your left hand on your thigh
   a) Your right foot should be directly beneath your arm, while your left foot (leg) should be angled outward
3) Inhale and brace your core (posterior pelvic tilt)
4) Rotate your torso so your left shoulder is turned down toward the floor and push your hips to the right
   a) Most of your weight should now be on your left leg
5) Turn your head and look up at your right hand
6) Lean to the side, slide your left hand down your leg, and try to keep your right leg straight, bending your left leg only slightly, exhaling slowly
7) Lean as far down as you can while reaching down your leg, go about halfway down the shin
   a) You should feel a stretch in the back of your left leg and the right side of your torso
   b) Focus on keeping your right hand pointed up toward the ceiling
8) Hold for 1-3 seconds and stand up, untwisting your torso as you do so
   a) Keep your right hand overhead and your left hand against your leg as you stand up
9) Repeat for the desired number of repetitions and then switch sides

Make it easier: Bring the arm down from overhead, don't bend as far

Make it harder: Hold for up to 10 seconds, hold a weight in the hand overhead

Standing Torso Twist

Muscles worked: Rectus abdominis, transverse abdominis, hip flexors, latissimus dorsi, erector spinae, pectoralis major

Be careful if: You have low- or mid-back issues

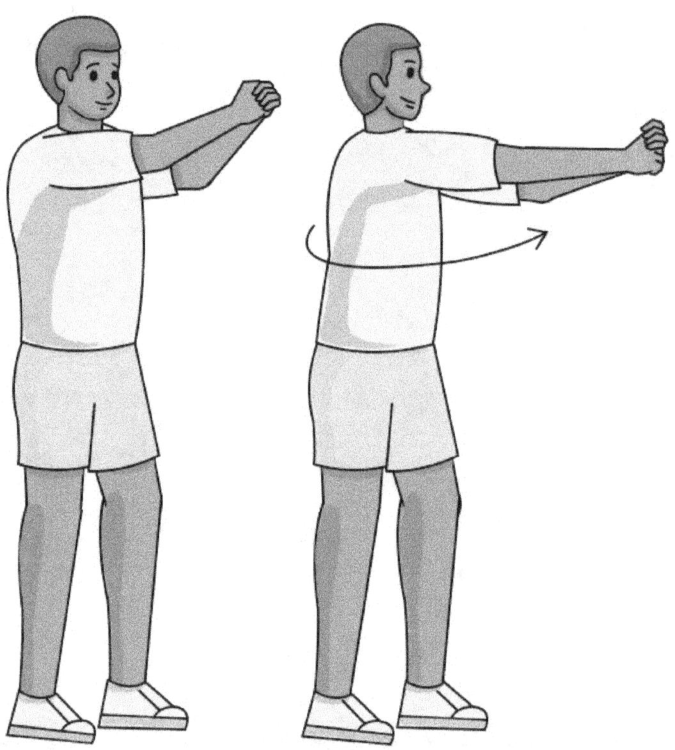

1) Stand upright and tall, feet about shoulder-width apart, toes turned out slightly
   a) You can stand with your back against a wall or counter for some added stability
2) Clasp your hands in front of you or place them on your hips
3) Inhale and brace your core (posterior pelvic tilt)
4) Slowly twist to the right and hold for 1-3 seconds, and exhale
5) Inhale as you come back to center and twist in the opposite direction

Make it easier: Brace a little less, don't twist as much

Make it harder: Press your palms together further engaging your core, hold for up to 10 seconds, lift the opposing knee as the direction you are twisting

Front to Back Rock

Muscles worked: Calves, hamstrings, quadriceps, rectus abdominis, transverse abdominis, latissimus dorsi, erector spinae

Be careful if: You have ankle, knee, hip, low-back, or shoulder issues

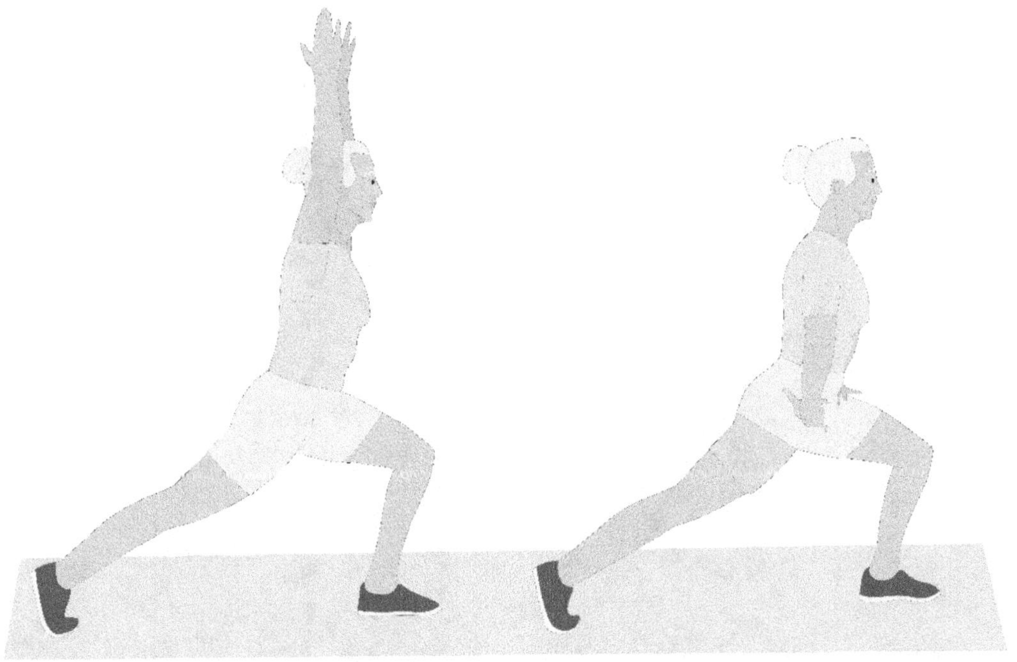

1. Stand up tall, feet about shoulder-width apart with arms hanging at your sides
2. Inhale and brace your core (posterior pelvic tilt)
3. Step slightly forward on your right foot while swinging your arms forward and up overhead, exhaling slowly, hold for 1 second
4. Step backward carefully with the right foot and swing the arms down and back until your right foot is planted
5. Repeat for the desired number of repetitions and then switch sides

Make it easier: Move more slowly, do not put your arms up as high, place one hand on a wall or back of chair for stability, don't move your foot as far forward or backward

Make it harder: Step a little further forward and backward, move a little more quickly, alternate feet.

High to Low Woodchopper

Muscles worked: External/internal oblique, rectus abdominis, transverse abdominis, erector spinae, latissimus dorsi, hip flexors

Be careful if: You have shoulder, back, or hip issues

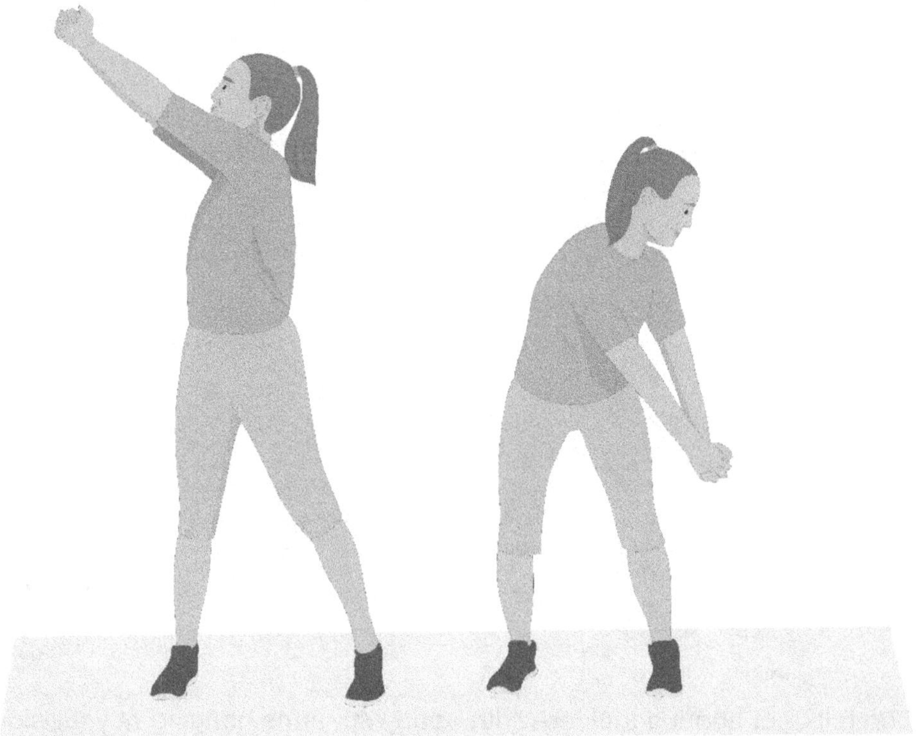

1) Stand tall with feet about shoulder-width apart, left foot slightly behind the right foot
   a) Stand against a wall for stability if need be
2) Clasp your hands together and extend them up overhead and across your body to the left
3) Inhale and brace your core (posterior pelvic tilt)
4) With almost straight arms, make a sweeping, chopping-like movement diagonally downward to the right
5) Hold for 1 second
6) Repeat for the desired number of repetitions and then switch sides, make sure the right foot comes slightly in front of the left foot this time

Make it easier: Raise one arm instead of both, do not twist so far

Make it harder: Brace more firmly, bend at the hip and "chop" down further

Standing Pelvic Tilt (Anterior & Posterior)

Muscles worked: Quadriceps, erector spinae, multifidus, quadratus lumborum, external/internal oblique, psoas (anterior), hamstring, quadriceps, gluteus maximus/medius, rectus abdominis, external/internal oblique (posterior)

Be careful if: You have low back issues

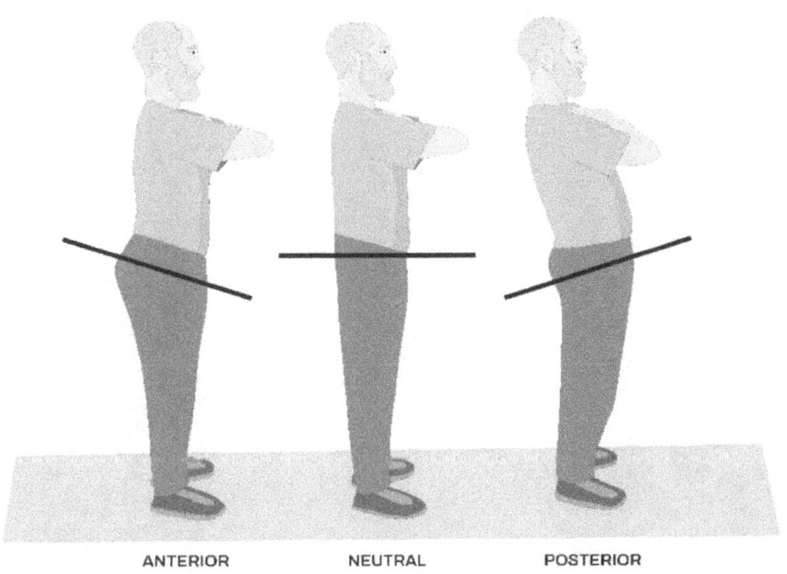

1) Stand up tall, feet about shoulder-width apart and flat on the floor
   a) Stand against a wall to get more feedback!
2) Place your hands on your hips

(Posterior Pelvic Tilt)
3) Inhale and slowly rock the top of your hips back and tuck your tailbone under, you'll feel yourself curling forward a bit
4) Hold for 1-3 seconds, exhaling slowly
   a) Note: As a visual aid, imagine your pelvis is functioning as a bowl full of water. During a posterior pelvic tilt you want to focus on tilting the bowl backwards so that water flows out of the bowl through your back. For an anterior tilt, the bowl will tilt forward and water will flow out the front.

(Anterior Pelvic Tilt)
5) Inhale and begin to reverse this motion
6) Exhale slowly and begin to slowly stick your tailbone "out" or behind you
7) Hold for 1-3 seconds

Make it easier: Don't move the pelvis as much

Make it harder: Hold for up to 10 seconds

Good Morning (also Forward Bend)

Muscles worked: Erector spinae, rectus abdominis, transverse abdominis, gluteus maximus, hip flexors

Be careful if: You have low-back issues

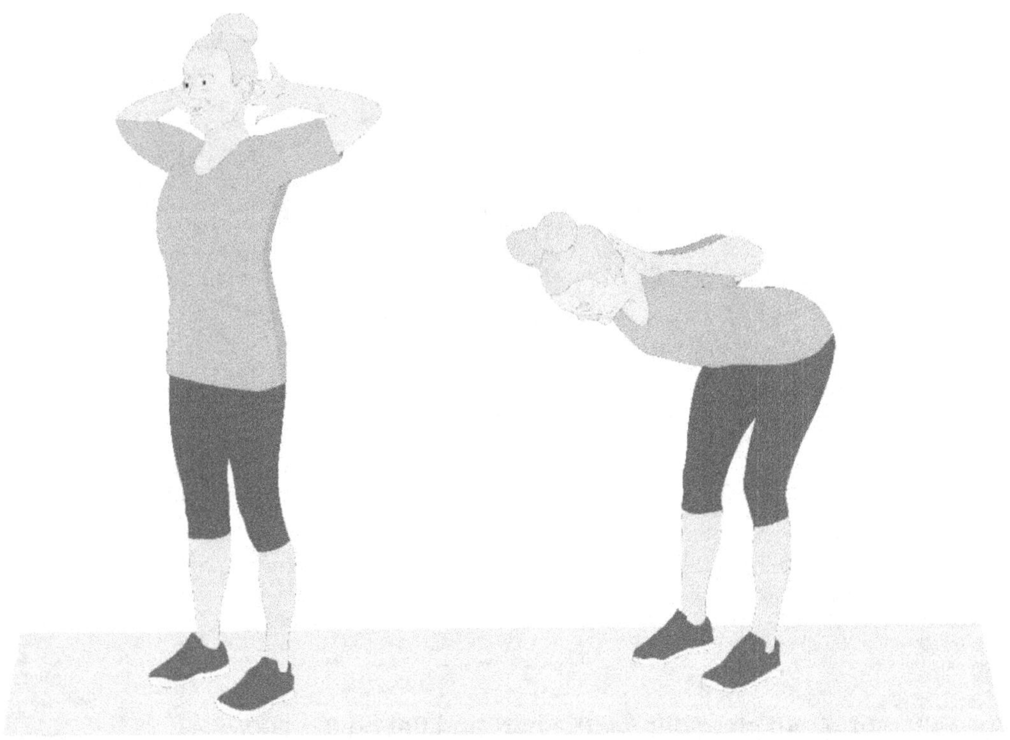

1) Stand up tall, feet about shoulder-width apart
2) Place your hands behind your ears, behind your head, or on your hips
   a) Do not pull on your head or neck
3) Inhale and brace your core (posterior pelvic tilt)
4) Slowly bend forward at the hip, moving your upper body as one single unit, exhaling slowly
   a) Only go as far forward as you feel comfortable
5) Pause for 1-3 seconds, squeeze your glutes, and return to an upright position

Make it easier: Place your hands on a counter or back of the chair to brace yourself as you lower, don't fold as far forward

Make it harder: Put your arms above your head, hold a small weight in front of your chest, bend further, hold for up to 10 seconds

Standing Side Crunch

Muscles worked: Rectus abdominis, transverse abdominis, hip flexors, erector spinae, psoas, quadratus lumborum, external/internal obliques, quadriceps

Be careful if: You have ankle, knee, hip, low-back, or shoulder issues

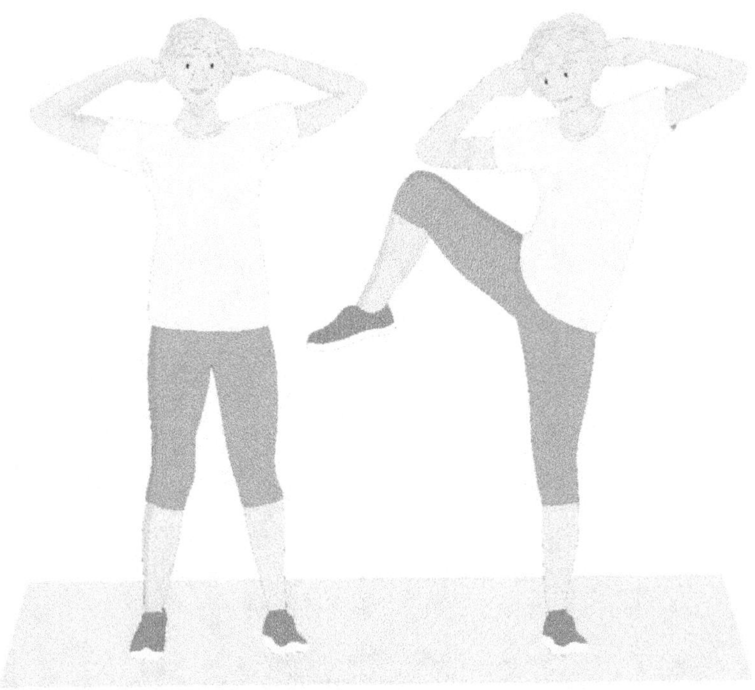

1) Stand up tall, feet about shoulder-width apart and toes turned out slightly
   a) You can stand with your back against a wall or counter for some added stability
2) Place your hands behind your ears or head, or even on your shoulders
   a) Do not pull on your head or neck
3) Inhale and brace your core (pelvic tilt)
4) Bend to the left slightly and lift your left knee up towards your left elbow, exhaling slowly
   a) Focus on moving your left knee out to the side and up rather than just straight up the front of your body
   b) Make sure your hips and shoulders remain square and facing forward, and your chest stays high
5) Hold for 1-3 seconds
6) Return your leg back to the ground, switch sides, and repeat

Make it easier: Don't bend as much, don't bring the knee as high or elbow so low

Make it harder: Hold for up to 10 seconds, bring the elbow and knee closer

Standing Figure 8 (or Standing Kayak Row)

Muscles worked: Latissimus dorsi, trapezius, rectus abdominis, transverse abdominis, external/internal obliques, erector spinae

Be careful if: You have shoulder, back, or hip issues

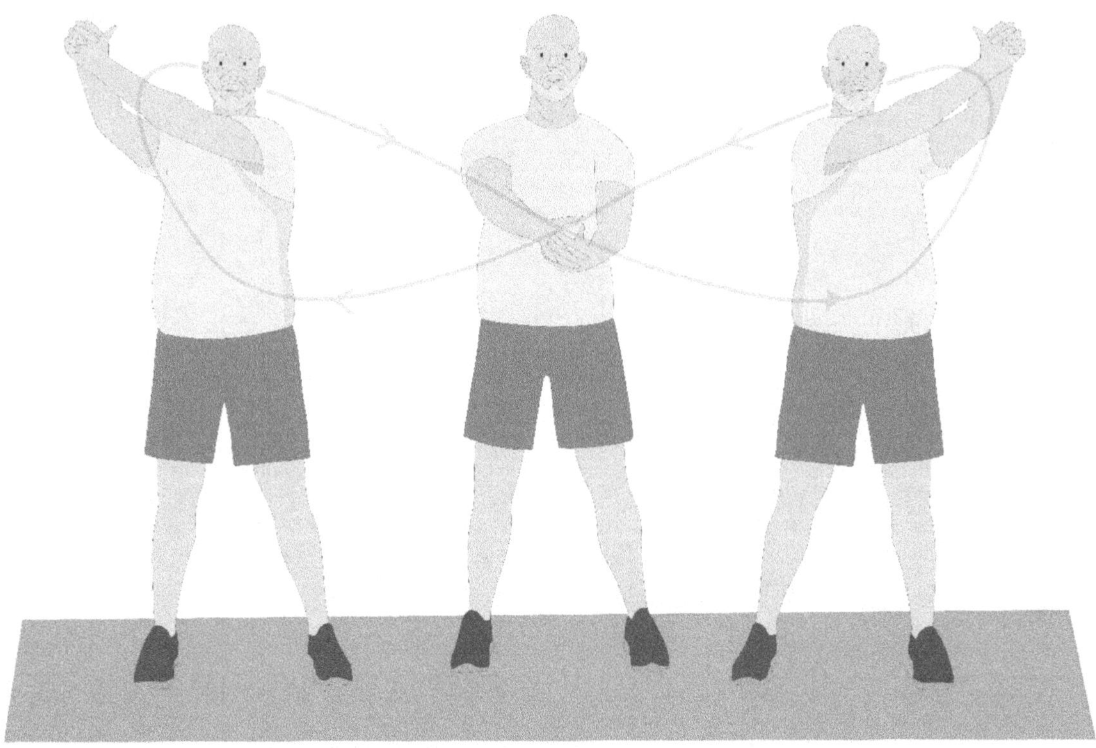

1) Stand upright and tall, feet about shoulder-width apart
   a) Stand against a wall for stability
2) Stack your forearms on top of one another
3) Inhale and brace your core (posterior pelvic tilt)
4) Begin to slowly make a figure 8 with your arms (or pretend you are paddling a kayak), exhaling slowly
5) Once back to the starting position, reverse the motion
   a) Twist at the waist and remain upright the entire time

Make it easier: Clasp your hands together, keeping elbows at your side, make a smaller figure 8, don't twist as much

Make it harder: Make the figure 8 large, extend your arms out in front to exaggerate the movement, lift one foot off of the ground

Hip Circles

Muscles worked: Rectus abdominis, transverse abdominis, external/internal oblique, hip flexors, gluteus maximus

Be careful if: You have low-back or hip issues

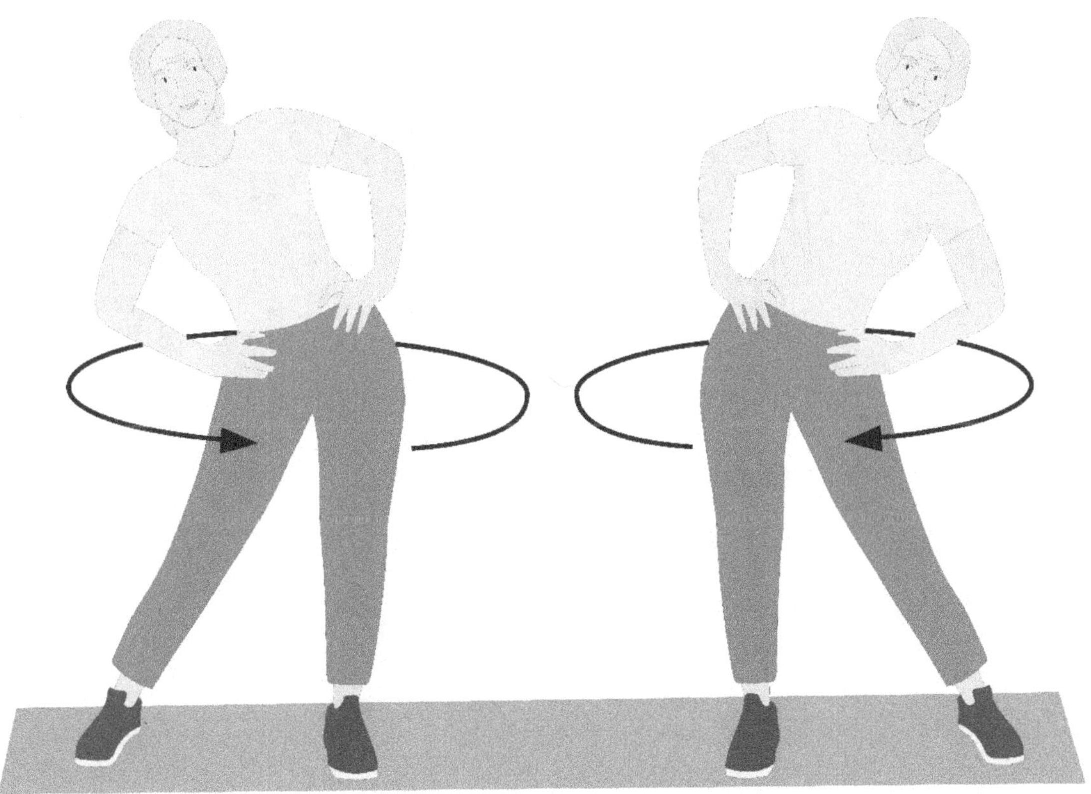

1) Stand upright and tall, feet about shoulder-width apart
2) Place your hands behind your ears, behind your head, or on your hips
   a) Do not pull on your head or neck
3) Inhale and brace your core (pelvic tilt)
4) Slowly push your right hip out until most of your weight is on the right leg, slowly lean backward as you push the hip forward and to the left
5) Continue making this circle slowly, until you have completed a full counter clockwise circle
6) Reverse this motion and create a circle going clockwise

Make it easier: Make your circle smaller, place your hands on a counter or back of chair to brace yourself

Make it harder: Pick one foot up off of the ground, make your circle larger

Standing Side Bend

Muscles worked: External/internal obliques, transverse abdominals, rectus abdominis, quadratus lumborum

Be careful if: You have low-back issues

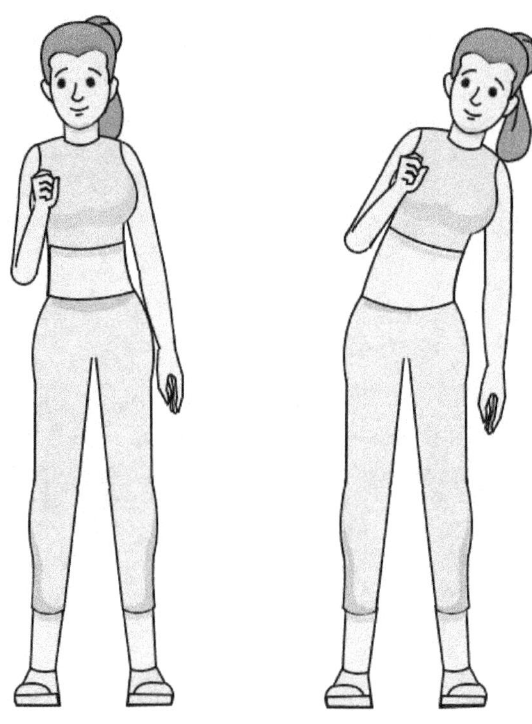

1) Stand upright and tall, feet about shoulder-width apart
   a) Stand against a wall for stability
2) Inhale and brace your core (posterior pelvic tilt)
3) Lean slowly to your left as far as you comfortably can, exhaling slowly
4) Hold for 1-3 seconds
5) Return back upright, switch sides, and repeat

Make it easier: Don't lean as far, hold on to the back of a chair or countertop

Make it harder: Hold for up to 10 seconds, put arms up in the air or out to your sides, hold weight in your hands, lift one foot off of the ground

Standing Bicycle Crunch

Muscles worked: External/internal obliques, rectus abdominis, transverse abdominis, hip flexors, quadriceps, hamstrings

Be careful if: You have hip, low-, or mid-back issues

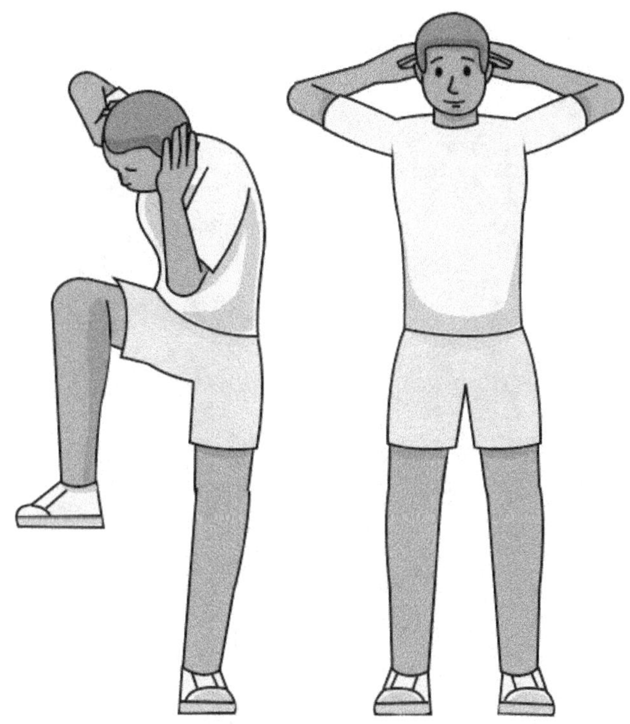

1) Stand upright and tall, feet about shoulder-width apart
    a) Stand against a wall for stability
2)   Inhale and brace your core (posterior pelvic tilt)
3) Slowly pull your left knee towards your head and reach your right elbow towards the knee, exhaling slowly
    a) The elbow and knee do not have to touch, get them as close together as you can without pain or discomfort
4) Hold for 1-3 seconds
5) Return to start, switch legs and arms, and repeat

Make it easier: Reach with your hand instead of your elbow, don't lift the knee as high

Make it harder: Touch the elbow to the knee

Sumo Side Crunch

Muscles worked: Gluteus maximus, adductors, external/internal obliques, quadriceps, hamstrings, transverse abdominis, rectus abdominis, hip flexors, calves

Be careful if: You have hip, low-back, or shoulder issues

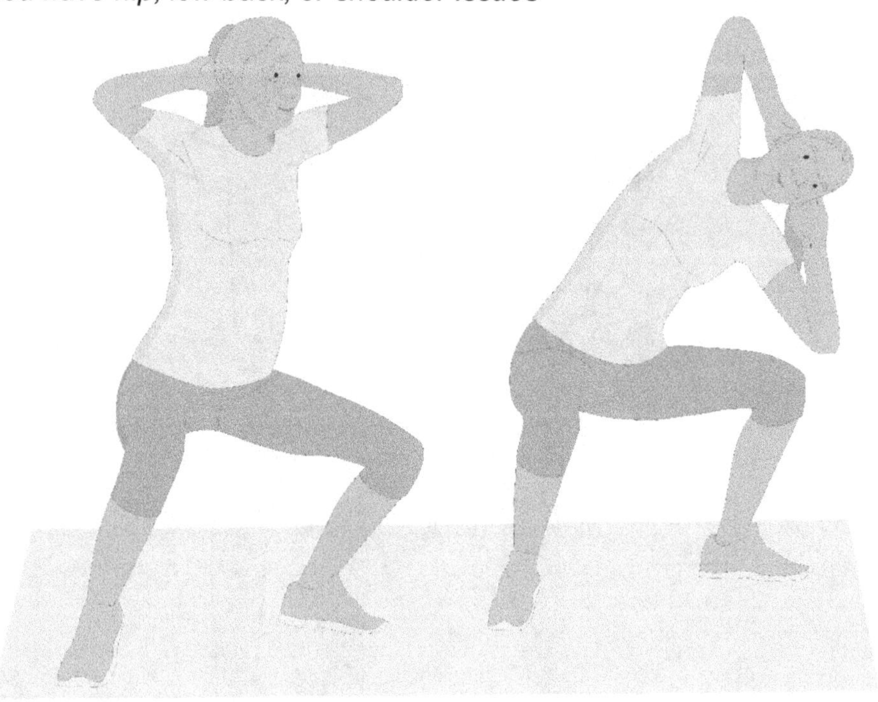

1) Stand upright and tall, feet wide (like a Sumo wrestler), knees bent slightly, toes pointing outwards
   a) Stand against a wall for stability
2) Place your hands behind your ears, behind your head, or on your hips
   a) Do not pull on your head or neck
3) Inhale and brace your core (posterior pelvic tilt)
4) Slowly tilt towards your left side, exhaling slowly
5) Hold for 1-3 seconds
6) Return back to start, switch sides, and repeat

Make it easier: Don't place your feet as wide, don't tilt as far, leave arms by your sides

Make it harder: Hold for up to 10 seconds, bend your knees further

Standing core exercises are a great way to build core strength. As previously mentioned, they are a great functional way to challenge your core musculature in a way that you would on any given day as you move about and live your life. Many of these exercises mimic what your body would be doing if you were to go up a flight or even one stair, if you were to bend to pick something up, if you needed to reach across your body, or even to take a step backward or forward. Another benefit of standing core exercise is you can add a modicum of safety by standing against a wall or near a countertop or chair before needing to do these exercises seated. It is a myth that you are "cheating" if you have your fingertips or hand on something for stability as you perform these exercises. In fact, it's often best to take the safer route so you can receive greater benefit from the exercise in and of itself. It's better that you get the strength training to increase your balance and stability with the hopes that one day you may not have to hold on!

Chapter 11 – Total Body Exercises

As you have perused this book, hopefully, you have gleaned that the core is a part of every move we perform, exercise-related or not. Total body exercises can be a great way to target your core and strengthen the rest of your body, essentially giving you a bit more bang for your buck. Also, there is an inherent functionality of total body exercises and the core. They come into play as there aren't many other modes of exercising that can really mimic what we do each and every day, outside of total body exercises, especially ones that focus on how to control your own body weight as you move! Total body exercises focus on improved mobility and control over your entire body. Moving through these exercises in a stable and controlled way will help your brain and muscles work in unison during other simple tasks. Total body exercise also carries many other exciting benefits including burning more calories in a single session, making it a time saver and ideal for home workouts. You could even get away with less workout sessions per week, meaning more time for recovery and other things you enjoy!

These, characteristically, will act as a routine on their own. If you already strength train regularly be mindful of where you add these in as you'll need to give your muscles time to recover. However, if you don't already have a strength training program, feel free to perform these exercises anywhere from 2-4 days per week, leaving a bare minimum of 24 hours for rest and recovery in between. If you haven't exercised in a while, you might even consider 48 hours between sessions because you could be a little sore or stiff. If you're still sore by the time your next workout rolls around that's okay. Exercising sore muscles can help get rid of some of that lactic acid and get fresh oxygen to your muscles. Just listen to your body and don't do anything that's painful.

Perform one to three sets of each exercise you choose. Aim for 8-12 quality repetitions of each. You can break these repetitions up if you need to, or make the repetition range a goal.

Suitcase Carry

Muscles worked: Rectus abdominis, transverse abdominis, erector spinae, quadratus lumborum, external/internal obliques, trapezius, latissimus dorsi, deltoids, biceps, triceps, forearms, hands

Be careful if: You have upper-back or shoulder issues

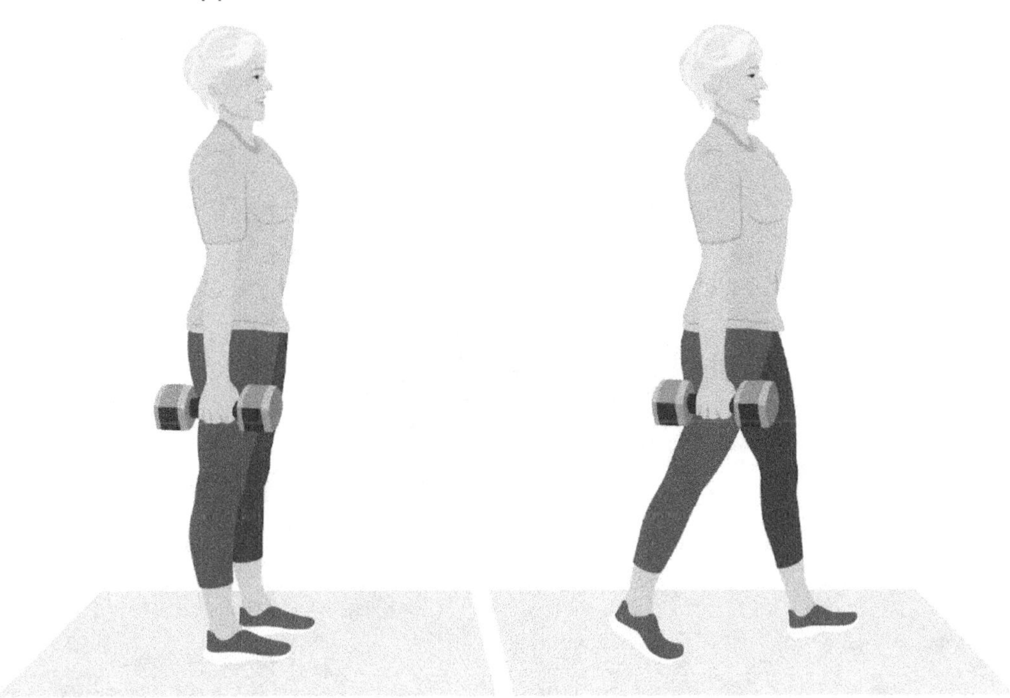

1) Stand upright and tall, feet about shoulder-width apart
   a) You can stand next to a wall or counter for some added stability
2) You should have one weight in your left hand
   a) This weight should be challenging but not so heavy you feel you will fall
3) Inhale and brace your core (posterior pelvic tilt)
4) Very slowly begin to walk about 20-25 yards, exhaling slowly
   a) Make sure your hips and shoulders remain square and facing forward and your chest and head stay high
   b) Imagine a glass of water on your head you don't want to fall off
5) Once you have gone your distance, switch the weight to the right hand and head back to start

Make it easier: Hold a lighter weight, march in place, or stand on one foot

Make it harder: Hold a heavier weight, walk a bit faster or further

Squat

Muscles worked: Quadriceps, hamstrings, gluteus maximus, rectus abdominis, transverse abdominis, erector spinae, calves

Be careful if: You have ankle, knee, hip, or low-back issues

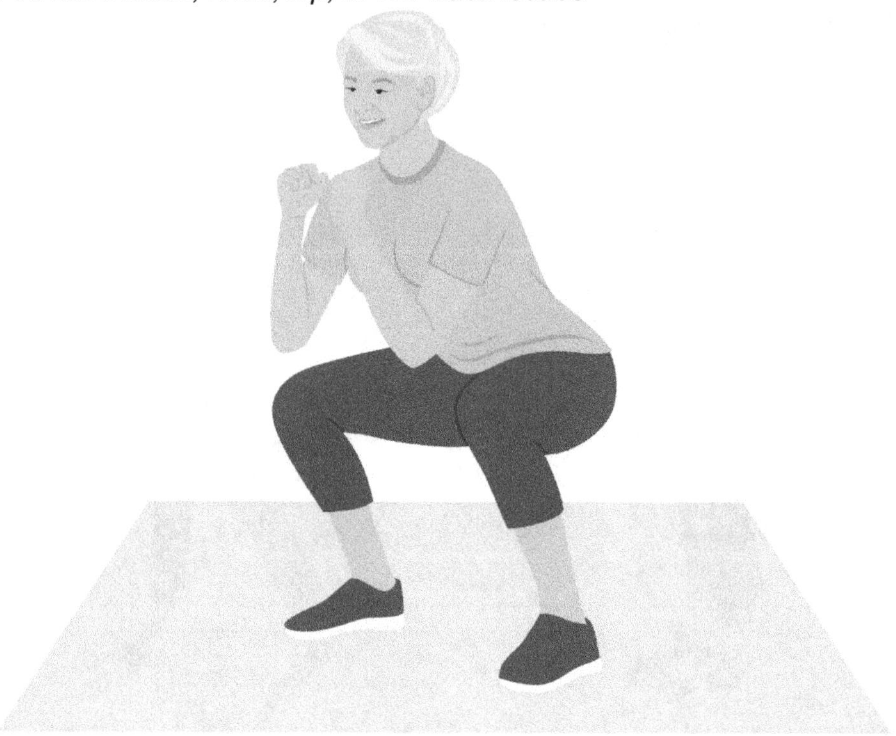

1) Stand with feet slightly wider than hip-width apart, toes turned slightly outward
   a) This ensures your knees do not bow, toes and knees should all point the same direction
   b) You can also set your legs up wide to target the inner thigh
2) Place your hands on your hips or hold them out in front, look straight ahead of you and keep your chest upright.
3) Inhale and brace your core (posterior pelvic tilt), start to shift your weight back into your heels while pushing your hips behind you as you squat down
   a) Think about pointing your tailbone between your heels
4) Continue to lower yourself until your thighs are almost parallel to the floor (knees at a 90 degree angle) or you're unable to keep your chest up.
5) Hold for 1-3 seconds
   a) Your feet should remain flat on the ground, and your knees should remain over your second toe (by the way, it's ok if your knees go over your toes!)
6) Exhale as you push through your feet and back up to standing

Make it easier: Don't bend your knees as much, place your hands on a countertop or use suspension straps to help you down and up, use a chair to begin from or go down to.

Make it harder: Hold for up to 10 seconds, hold a weight in your hands, add a small jump or explode upward

Deadlift

Muscles worked: Hamstrings, gluteus maximus, erector spinae, multifidus, hip flexors, rectus abdominis, transverse abdominis, erector spinae, trapezius, latissimus dorsi

Be careful if: You have ankle, knee, hip, or low-back issues

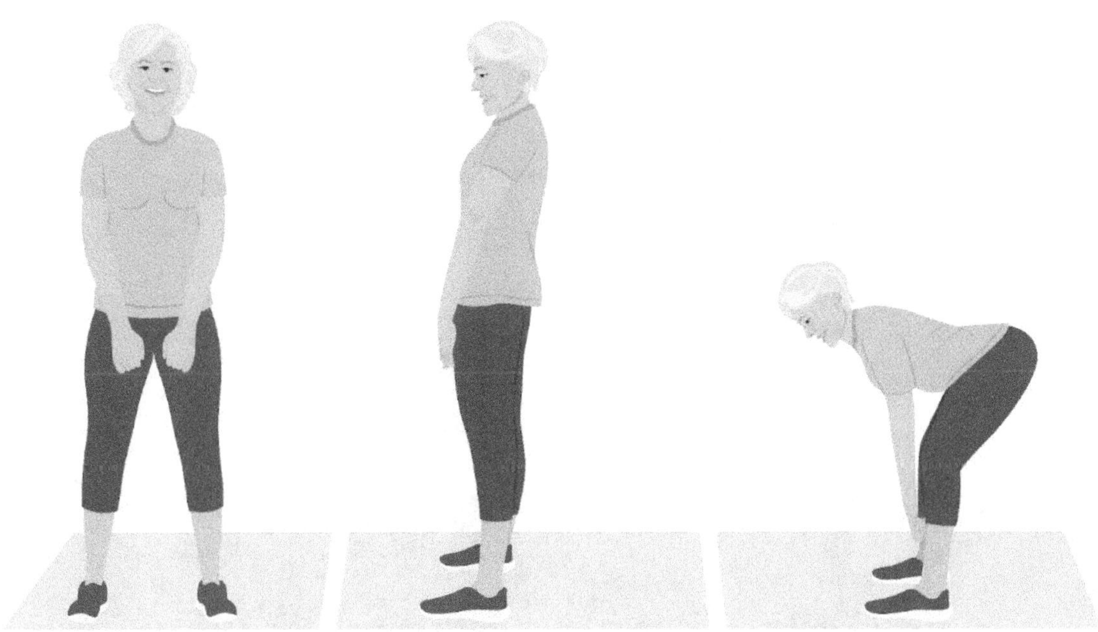

1) Stand upright and tall, feet about shoulder-width apart, toes pointing forward, knees slightly bent
   a) You can stand near a wall or counter for some added stability
2) Arms will remain by your sides, place your hands on your thighs, bring your shoulders back and down a bit
   a) This "packs your back", meaning your upper back muscles encompass your spine and protect it by providing stability. This will also ensure your upper body stays stiff and moves as one unit
3) Inhale and brace your core (posterior pelvic tilt)
4) Push back with the hips and let your hands travel down your legs as you do this, exhaling slowly
   a) Stop when you feel a pull in the hamstrings
   b) No need to go much past halfway down your lower leg
5) Hold for 1-3 seconds
6) Squeeze your glutes (butt) and return back to an upright position, reset and repeat

Make it easier: Don't bend as far

Make it harder: Hold on to weight, bend as far as you can maintaining a neutral spine

Kickstand Deadlift (also B-Stance Deadlift)

Muscles worked: Hamstrings, gluteus maximus, erector spinae, multifidus, hip flexors, rectus abdominis, transverse abdominis, erector spinae, trapezius, latissimus dorsi

Be careful if: You have ankle, knee, hip, or low-back issues

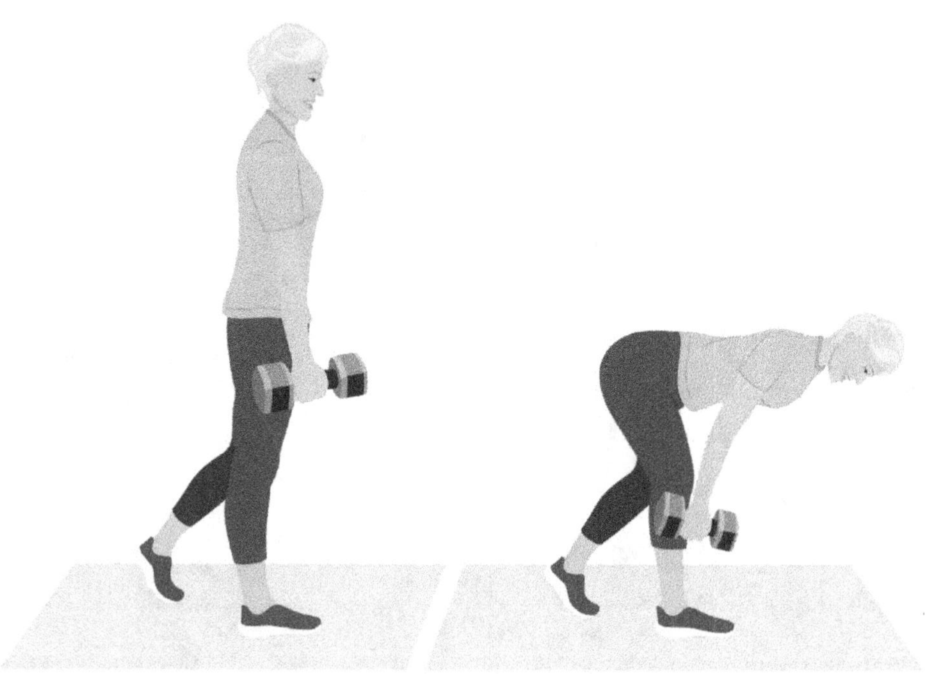

1) Stand upright and tall, feet about shoulder width apart, toes pointing forward, bring your left foot just behind you, toe on the ground (like a kickstand)
   a) You can stand near a wall or counter for some added stability
2) Arms will remain by your sides, place your right hand on your right thigh, bring your shoulders back and down a bit (squeeze your shoulder blades together) and hold them that way through the entire movement.
   a) Think about "packing your back" again just like with the traditional deadlift.
3) Inhale and brace your core (pelvic tilt)
4) Push back with the hips and let your hands travel down your legs as you do this, exhaling slowly
   a) Stop when you feel a pull in the hamstrings
   b) No need to go much past halfway down your lower leg
5) Hold for 1-3 seconds
6) Squeeze your glutes (butt) and return back to an upright position, reset and repeat

Make it easier: Don't bend forward as much

Make it harder: Hold for up to 10 seconds, hold weight in one or both hands

Hand Elevated Push Up

Muscles worked: Rectus abdominis, transverse abdominis, hip flexors, erector spinae, psoas, quadratus lumborum, external/internal obliques, quadriceps

Be careful if: You have ankle, knee, hip, low-back, or shoulder issues

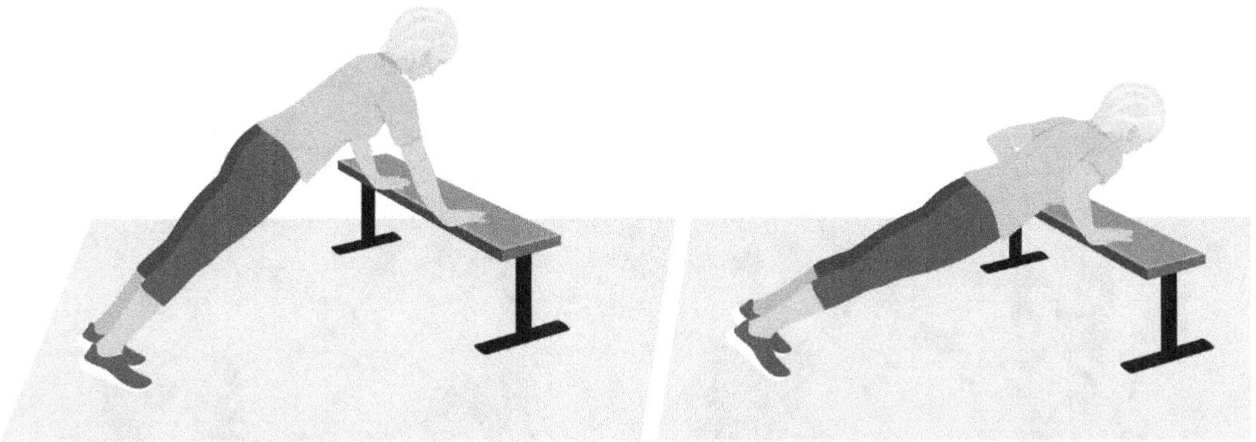

1) Find an elevated surface such as a countertop, back of a couch, back of a chair, dining room table, or wall
   a) Make sure this surface is stable.
2) Hands should be shoulder width apart, and the heels of your hand are in-line with your shoulders.
3) Inhale and brace your core (posterior pelvic tilt)
4) Begin to lower yourself towards your hands, look just past the fingertips to keep a neutral neck
5) Keeping your elbows around a 45° angle (at most), come as far down as you can without pain or discomfort, exhaling slowly
   a) You should feel your shoulders blades coming together when you're at the bottom of this movement, and come back apart as you push away.
6) Hold for 1-3 seconds.
7) Push through your hands and back up and repeat
   a) Your whole body should move as one unit up and down

Make it easier: Find a higher surface for your hands, don't lower yourself as far

Make it harder: Hold for up to 10 seconds, find a lower surface for your hands

Surrenders

Muscles worked: Rectus abdominis, transverse abdominis, hip flexors, erector spinae, quadratus lumborum, external/internal obliques, quadriceps, hamstrings, gluteus maximus, trapezius, latissimus dorsi

Be careful if: You have ankle, knee, hip, back, or shoulder issues

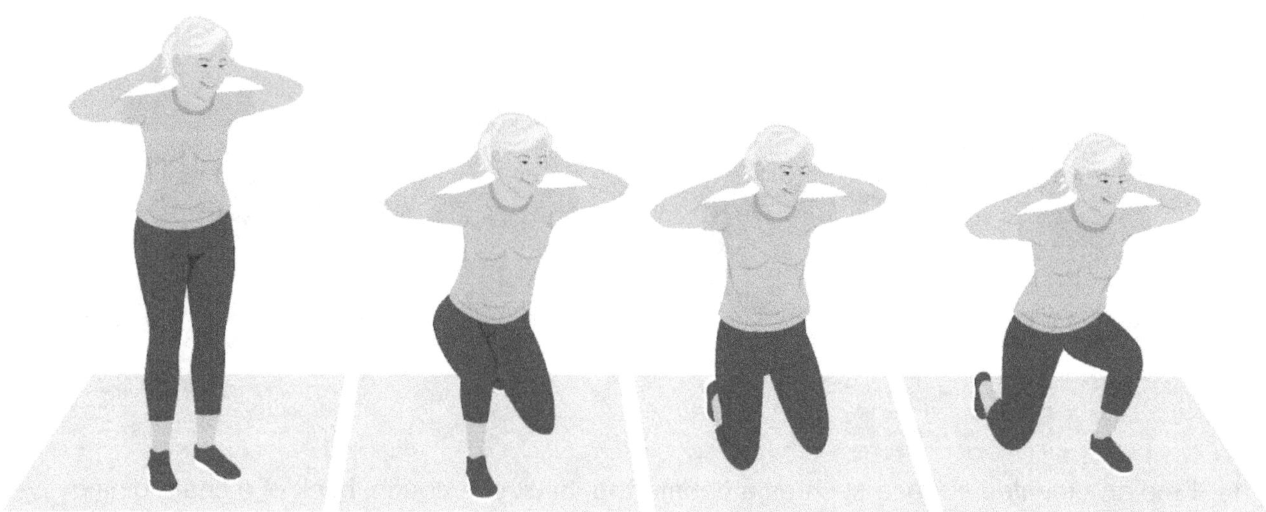

1) Stand upright and tall, feet about shoulder width apart, toes turned out slightly on a mat or other soft surface
    a) You can stand near a wall or counter for some added stability
2) Place your hands behind your ears, behind your head, or on your shoulders
    a) Do not pull on your head or neck
3) Inhale and brace your core (posterior pelvic tilt)
4) Bring your left knee to the ground, and then your right, exhaling slowly
    a) Make sure your hips and shoulders remain square and facing forward and your chest stays high
5) Return to start by bringing your left knee up and then your right back to standing
6) Switch the lead leg to the right and repeat
    a) Keep your body as still as possible as you move throughout

Make it easier: Kneel on something higher such as a rolled-up blanket or towel, place your hands on a countertop for assistance, bring one knee down and back instead of both knees down

Make it harder: Raise your hands above your head, maintain a squat position instead of standing upright, hold weight in front of your chest

Waiters Carry

Muscles worked: Rectus abdominis, transverse abdominis, erector spinae, quadratus lumborum, external/internal obliques, trapezius, latissimus dorsi, deltoids, biceps, triceps, forearms, hands

Be careful if: You have upper-back or shoulder issues

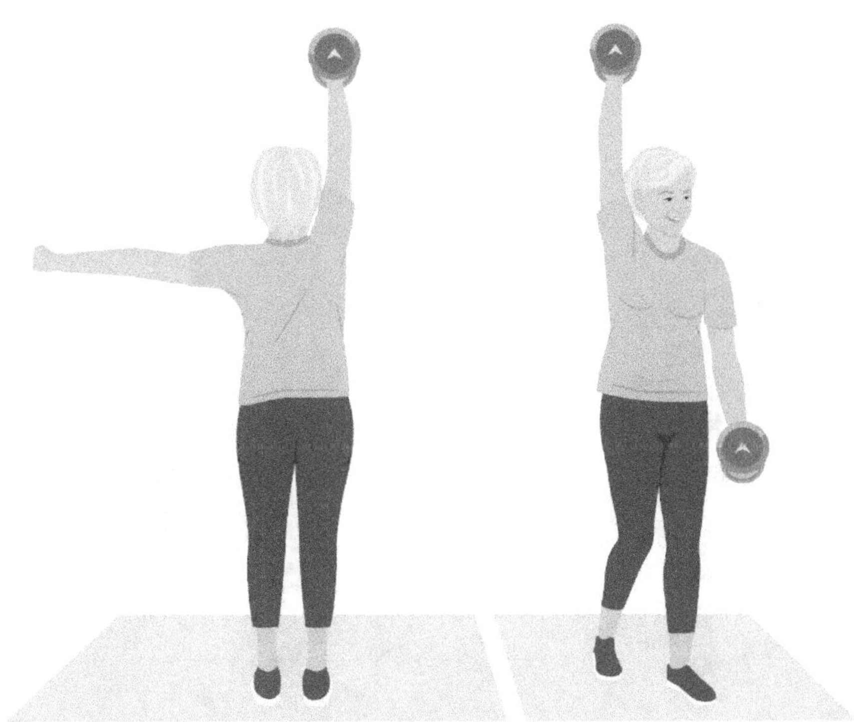

1) Stand upright and tall, feet about shoulder width apart
    a) You can stand next to a wall or counter for some added stability
2) You should have one weight in your left hand
    a) This weight should be challenging but not so heavy you can't lift it overhead
3) Inhale and brace your core (posterior pelvic tilt) and bring the weight overhead carefully
4) Very slowly begin to walk about 20-25 yards, exhaling slowly
    a) Make sure your hips and shoulders remain square and facing forward and your chest and head stay high
    b) Imagine a glass of water on your head you don't want to fall off
5) Once you have gone your distance, switch the weight to the right hand and head back to start

Make it easier: Hold a lighter weight or none at all, march in place, or stand on one foot

Make it harder: Hold a heavier weight, walk a bit faster or further, have a weight in each hand

Farmers Carry

Muscles worked: Rectus abdominis, transverse abdominis, erector spinae, quadratus lumborum, external/internal obliques, trapezius, latissimus dorsi, deltoids, biceps, triceps, forearms, hands

Be careful if: You have upper-back or shoulder issues

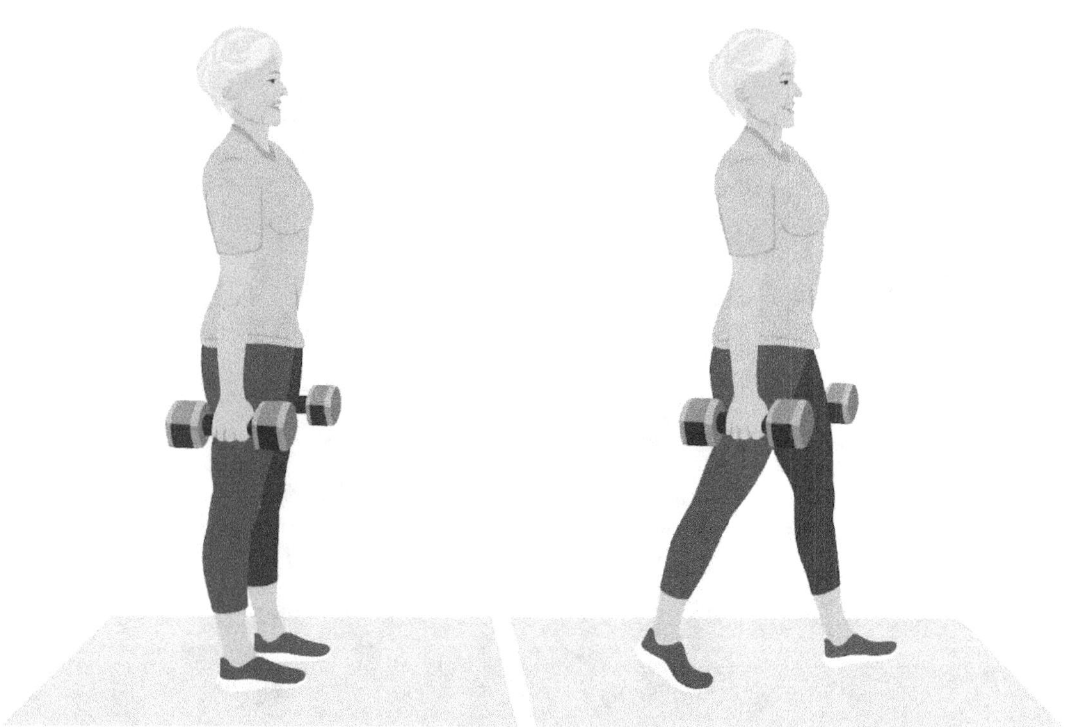

1) Stand upright and tall, feet about shoulder width apart
   a) You can stand next to a wall or counter for some added stability
2) You should have a weight in both hands
   a) This weight should be challenging but not so heavy you feel you will fall
3) Inhale and brace your core (pelvic tilt)
4) Very slowly begin to walk about 20-25 yards, exhaling slowly
   a) Make sure your hips and shoulders remain square and facing forward and your chest and head stay high
   b) Imagine a glass of water on your head you don't want to fall off
5) Once you have gone your distance, turn around back to start

Make it easier: Hold a lighter weight, march in place, or stand on one foot

Make it harder: Hold a heavier weight, walk a bit faster or further

Bent Over Row

Muscles worked: Rectus abdominis, transverse abdominis, hip flexors, erector spinae, trapezius, latissimus dorsi

Be careful if: You have hip, low-back, or shoulder issues

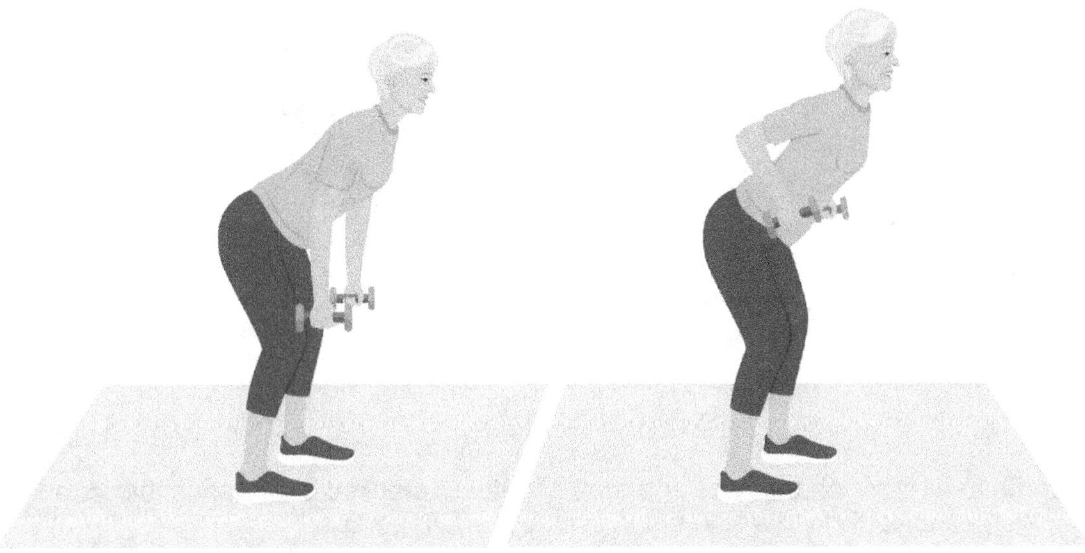

1) Stand upright and tall, feet about shoulder-width apart, toes turned out slightly
   a) You can stand near a wall or counter for some added stability
2) Let your arms rest by your sides and bring your shoulders back and down a bit
   a) This "packs your back" just like with the deadlifts mentioned above.
3) Bend at the hip to around a 45° angle and let your arms hang towards the ground
4) Inhale and brace your core (posterior pelvic tilt)
5) Drive your elbows straight back and squeeze the shoulder blades together, exhaling slowly
6) Hold for 1-3 seconds
7) Return arms back to start and repeat

Make it easier: Don't bend as far forward, don't drive the elbow back as far

Make it harder: Hold for up to 10 seconds, hold weight in each hand, bend up to 90° angle at the hip

Bear Squat

Muscles worked: Rectus abdominis, transverse abdominis, hip flexors, erector spinae, quadratus lumborum, external/internal obliques, quadriceps, hamstrings, deltoids, gluteus maximus, trapezius, latissimus dorsi, biceps, triceps, calves

Be careful if: You have ankle, knee, hip, back, shoulder, elbow, or wrist issues

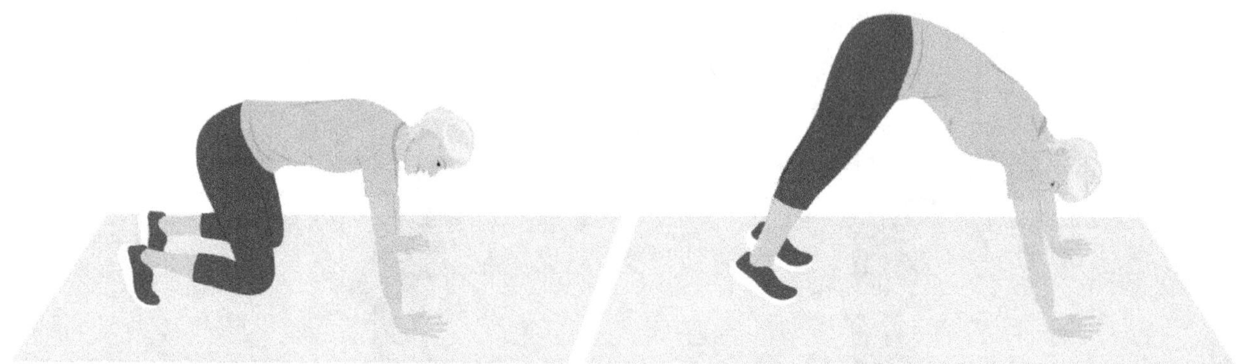

1. Come to all fours on the floor or a mat, shoulders stacked over hands, hips stacked over knees, keep your gaze a little out in front of your fingertips
2. Inhale and brace your core by performing a slight pelvic tilt (tuck your tailbone a bit) and draw your shoulder blades together
3. Lift your knees off of the ground a few inches (the lower the more challenging), exhaling slowly
4. Hold 1-3 seconds
5. Maintaining a straight line from your head to your tailbone, straighten your legs, then bend them back again so your knees are floating above the ground and repeat

Make it easier: Place your hands on an elevated surface such as a bench, chair or coffee table, don't hold for so long, leave one knee on the ground and alternate which legs straightens

Make it harder: Hold for up to 10 seconds, elevate the feet

Be careful during these movements, especially if you're new to fitness. While not inherently dangerous they do take a fair amount of cooperation through many different body parts to work properly. If you are unsure, choose a portion of the movement and practice that until you feel comfortable, then work on building upon that. You will still gain benefit and are less likely to injure yourself in the long run. Most, if not all, of these exercises mimic what you may perform on a day to day basis and can be your go-to for not only core strengthening but total body strengthening as well. Sprinkle in a few other core strength moves and you'll really benefit!

Many of these exercises can be adapted for nearly anyone. As long as you feel safe and confident, you can change things up a bit. However, it is best to err on the side of caution and check to make sure you are doing a movement correctly. With every other exercise out there, what you put into this is what you will get out of it!

Chapter 12 – Falls and Fall Risk Prevention

We all fall. It's one of those things in life that become rather pesky, but can turn into something debilitating or even life-threatening. There are obstacles all around us and while there's no 100% guaranteed way to keep you on your feet, there are a number of ways to help safeguard yourself, limiting the risk of serious injury if you do fall.

According to the CDC, in the United States, one in four adults ages 65 and older report falling each year. While not all falls result in an injury, about 37% of those who fall reported an injury that required medical treatment or restricted their activity for at least one day, resulting in an estimated nine million fall injuries. And those are just the reported ones.

Falls are the leading cause of injury-related death among adults ages 65 and older, and the fall death rate is increasing. The age-adjusted fall death rate increased by 41% from 55.3 per 100,000 in 2012 to 78 per 100,000 in 2021.

Falls among adults ages 65 and older are exceptionally costly. Each year, about ***$50 billion*** is spent on medical costs related to older adult falls—fatal injuries total $754 million, and the remainder is attributed to non-fatal fall injuries.

Non-fatal Falls
- $29 billion is paid by Medicare
- $12 billion is paid by private or out-of-pocket payers
- $9 billion is paid by Medicaid59

Falls are a very serious matter and can be incredibly costly. About 20% of falls result in a broken bone or head injury, and each year, around 300,000 individuals are hospitalized because of a hip fracture. Nearly all of which are caused by falls, 93%! Falls are the most common cause of traumatic brain injury as well and can lead to severe disability or death. Another cause for concern is when those falls lead to fear, injury, or disability, which, in a lot of cases, leads to loneliness, isolation, and decreased physical activity. It's a fact that when people fall, they often become scared they may fall again. This will often limit many of their actions so as not to fall again. Loneliness and isolation have a much more significant impact on physical and mental health than most realize (CDC, 2023). Those who are isolated or lonely are 50% more likely to die prematurely than their peers who are able to remain social (Psychology Today, 2019).

These statistics and numbers are pretty compelling, but what makes us more at risk of a fall? It's really a question of when we'll fall rather than if. We're all bound to fall down at one point or another. While there are some aspects of your environment that you can't control, luckily there are far more conditions that ARE within your control to prevent falls from happening as frequently. In turn, this keeps you safe, healthy, and happy while achieving a high quality of living. These conditions are often referred to as *risk factors*.

The risk factors you don't necessarily have any control over include;
- Age (no kidding!)
- Biological gender

According to the WHO, men typically have a higher incidence of death resulting from a fall. This could be due to lifestyle and gender differences. For example, a fall off a roof while cleaning gutters. Worldwide, males consistently sustain higher death rates and loss of ADL's than women from falls (WHO, 2021).

- Occupation
- Genetic predisposition to certain health issues that can lead to greater fall risk
- Diabetes
- Cardiovascular disease
- Socioeconomic factors

The most common risk factors you have control over are (CDC, Queensland Government):
- Lower body weakness
- Vitamin D deficiency (not enough vitamin D in your system)
- Difficulties with walking and balance
- Mismanagement of medications
  - taking them at the wrong time
  - taking them intermittently or not at all
- Medications
  - tranquilizers
  - antidepressants
  - sedatives
  - Opioids and other pain killers
  - some over-the-counter medications, among others
- Vision problems
- Foot pain, poor footwear, or improperly worn footwear
- Inadequate sleep or rest
- Poor nutrition
- Inattention to outdoor hazards
  - insufficient light
  - high curbs or curb height changes
  - broken or cracked sidewalks
  - roots or rocks
  - icy, wet, mossy, leaf or plant debris strewn walkways or sidewalks
  - yard tools left out or hoses across the ground
- Inattention to indoor hazards
  - insufficient light
  - throw rugs without an anti-slip mat underneath
  - cluttered floors or walkways from art, shoes, clothing, or pet toys
  - electrical cords

- flooring height changes
      - getting up at night without enough light
      - stepping over pets instead of making them move
  - Pets
      - we often don't want to disturb our furry friends but they are very unpredictable and are a leading cause of falls for those who own pets
  - Moving too quickly in general
      - to answer the phone or door
      - rushing to the bathroom because of incontinence
  - Use of alcohol or other intoxicants
  - Not using an appropriate mobility device or not using the device properly

Bear in mind it is very rarely only one of these risk factors. It's often a combination of these risk factors that increase the risk for a fall. Thankfully, there are several things you can do that will act as preventative maintenance to keep you from falling as often, and potentially no more! For instance, regular annual health exams are imperative! You can address numerous risk factors at once each year. Medical professionals can perform medication reviews, complete vision exams, update the status of chronic health conditions, and talk about strategies to maintain strength and balance. In addition, you can ask for referrals to a professional who can address any potential nutrition inadequacies or cognitive impairments you may not be aware of. You can make your home (indoor and outdoor) safer by removing scatter rugs, keeping clutter up off of the floor, making sure you have adequate light during all hours of the day, putting tools away, and removing or placing cords or hoses in safer out of the way places. You can limit the amount of recreational drugs or alcohol you consume, how much sleep you have, and you have a lot of control over your diet.

Last, and indisputably not least, staying active and strong! A Harvard Health contributor mentioned that core strength is vital for fall prevention, as your body's core is the epicenter from which every movement revolves. "As we walk, our bodies constantly have to adapt to ever-changing ground levels," says O'Neill. "Adequate core stability and strength help you better react to these sudden changes and prevent potential falls (Harvard Health). He isn't the only one who thinks so, this is a fact shared by top fitness professionals, doctors, scientists, and many others across the globe!

Understanding your current risk factors is the most important step you can take to reduce your chances of a fall. A very helpful tool created by the CDC is called the STEADI (Stopping Elderly Accidents, Deaths, and Injuries) tool. Here, you will find useful information on everything related to falls and fall risk for those over 65. There is information for providers but also for you! Access this information by going to www.cdc.gov/steadi.

The bottom line is that you will most likely fall once or more in your remaining years. Again, the great news is you have some control over how frequently that may be and how that fall will affect you. Core strength training is easily one of the most important factors in fall prevention, fall recovery (from a slip or almost fall), and recovery after a fall. With the numerous combinations of core strengthening exercises you have access to in this book, and with consistency in training, you will be setting yourself up for success in decreasing your risk for falls and helping to return to normal life if you do fall.

Conclusion

Let's recap some key concepts!

What is the core?
It is the first of the body's muscles to contract when we make any kind of movement. Our core is the scaffolding that holds our skeleton upright, and it helps to protect our spine and other organs.

What muscles comprise the core?
More than just what we'd traditionally refer to as "abs", our core is assisted by other muscles, including those from the upper body - the trapezius and latissimus dorsi, as well as lower body muscles such as the gluteus maximus, hamstrings, and quadriceps.

What does the core do?
Its primary function (outside of stabilization) is to help us breathe properly! Next up, it helps keep the spine unloaded as we move around and is the epicenter of our strength. To move well, our core must be strong and stable.

What are some advantages of a strong core and why should we do core exercises?
- Less falls and improved stability
- Quicker recovery from an injury or illness
- Joint support (from strong muscles)
- Increased energy
- Better sleep
- Less likely to suffer from issues such as diabetes, cardiovascular disease, sarcopenia, general weakness and instability
- Better bone density, less stress, anxiety, and depression
- Increased mobility, making social relationships like friendships and intimate partnerships easier
- Better able to travel
- Maintain independence and activities of daily living
- Less pain and discomfort

What can happen if you do not have a strong core?
All of those benefits may go away. Perhaps not completely, but enough to where your quality of life may not be as good as it could be.

What are the safety guidelines for exercising?
Warm-up and cool down, stretching, learning how to brace properly, being present as you exercise, making your muscles do the work, remembering to breathe properly, start slow and

increase the challenge gradually, listening to your body, being consistent, getting adequate rest, proper nutrition and hydration, and being aware of how hard you are working using an RPE (rate of perceived exertion) scale.

What are the signs and symptoms of a weak core?
- Poor posture
- Low-back pain
- You lack power and stability during everyday activities
- Discomfort when lying on your back
- Excessive inward or outward curvature of the spine
- Difficulty when standing from a squat or seated position
- You feel off-balance or unstable
- You have pain or discomfort in the pelvis
- You have difficulty walking upright without hunched shoulders.

Bear in mind these weaknesses do not have to be severe; they can be very mild symptoms, and if they are, this means you have caught things before they get worse!

Having an awareness of how your body moves
More notably, your spinal motion, pelvic motion, and shoulder motion. Knowing what these areas of the body feel like when moving is imperative to your brain connecting with your body in a powerful way. This better brain-body connection will ultimately result in a higher benefit from any and all exercises you do.

If you are able to learn and understand these concepts, you will have a great foundation for becoming stronger and more stable. Once you are able to put these concepts into practice and be consistent, you will be giving yourself the gift of stability, strength, and overall health that has far-reaching benefits. Sadly, many of the negatives that come from a weak core are so common they appear to be "normal".

If you believe you have the ability to make these positive changes to your life, you will become the exception, and that is truly what it means to honor yourself. We are given one body and one mind. There is no magic pill, there isn't one program that will solve your problems, and there is certainly not only one way to achieve these benefits. However, this book gives you the tools and knowledge to succeed. No matter where you are in life, no matter your current ability, mobility, or fitness level, you can make positive changes to your health and well-being that will lead to a better quality of life. In a world that may seem out of control, you have the power and ability to improve your core strength. Let's get started!

Thank You!

Thank you for your recent purchase! If you enjoyed this book, please consider writing a review. As a small business owner, this would mean the world!

Scanning the QR code above with your phone will take you directly to the Amazon review page

References

Erin V. Dorn, MS

CH 1
1. The real-world benefits of strengthening your core - Harvard Health
2. The Importance of Trunk Muscle Strength for Balance, Functional Performance, and Fall Prevention in Seniors: A Systematic Review | SpringerLink
3. Effects of core instability strength training on trunk muscle strength, spinal mobility, dynamic balance and functional mobility in older adults - PubMed (nih.gov)
4. https://agsjournals.onlinelibrary.wiley.com/doi/abs/10.1111/j.1532-5415.2000.tb03903.x
5. Core Composition and Function: The Core of 2014 Part 1 | Functional Movement Systems
6. https://brookbushinstitute.com/
7. Why Balance Training is NOT Core Stability Training (trainingpeaks.com)

CH 2
8. Core muscles and your posture | MS Trust (picture)
9. Osteoporosis | National Institute on Aging (nih.gov)
10. Economic Costs of Diabetes in the U.S. in 2017 - PubMed (nih.gov)
11. Health and Economic Costs of Chronic Diseases | CDC
12. The Medical Costs of Fatal Falls and Fall Injuries among Older Adults - PMC (nih.gov)

CH 3
13. Blood pressure chart: What your reading means - Mayo Clinic
14. Coronary artery disease - Symptoms and causes - Mayo Clinic
15. The Impact of Aerobic Exercise on HDL Quantity and Quality: A Narrative Review - PubMed (nih.gov)
16. Researchers link sedentary behavior to thinning in brain region critical for memory | UCLA
17. Sedentary behavior as a risk factor for cognitive decline? A focus on the influence of glycemic control in brain health - ScienceDirect
18. A1C test - Mayo Clinic
19. Blood Glucose & Exercise | ADA (diabetes.org)
20. Sarcopenia (Muscle Loss): Symptoms & Causes (clevelandclinic.org)

CH 4
21. The effect of duration of stretching of the hamstring muscle group for increasing range of motion in people aged 65 years or older - PubMed (nih.gov)
22. Dynamic vs. Static Stretching – Cleveland Clinic
23. 9 Benefits of Stretching: How to Start, Safety Tips, and More (healthline.com)
24. Benefits of massage therapy - Mayo Clinic Health System
25. Deep Breathing Benefits and How-To | Right as Rain (uwmedicine.org)
26. Stretching: Focus on flexibility - Mayo Clinic
27. Keeping good form when weight lifting | PureGym
28. Good Form vs. Bad Form: What You Don't Know (t-nation.com)
29. What It Actually Means to "Listen to Your Body" (greatist.com)
30. Sleep and Aging: What's Normal? | Johns Hopkins Medicine
31. How to Engage and Brace Your Core Quickly - Coach Sofia Fitness
32. To Achieve Big Goals, Start with Small Habits (hbr.org)
33. Protein Consumption and the Elderly: What Is the Optimal Level of Intake? - PubMed (nih.gov)

CH 5
34. Back pain - Symptoms and causes - Mayo Clinic

35. Low Back Pain: Causes, Diagnosis & Treatments (clevelandclinic.org)
36. Does trunk and hip muscles strength predict performance during a core stability test? - PubMed (nih.gov)
37. Curves of the Spine | Cedars-Sinai
38. Kyphosis | Cedars-Sinai
39. Squat for your life - ReActive Movement
40. Physical Inactivity: Physiological and Functional Impairments and Their Treatment | Musculoskeletal Key
41. Pelvic Floor Anatomy - Physiopedia (physio-pedia.com)
42. Pelvic Floor Dysfunction: Symptoms, Causes, and Treatment (healthline.com)
43. The Effects of Pelvic Floor Muscle Exercise Combined with Core Stability Exercise on Women with Stress Urinary Incontinence following the Treatment of Nonspecific Chronic Low Back Pain - PubMed (nih.gov)

CH 6
44. Supercharge Your Workout With This 3-Step Mental Preparation Protocol | BarBend
45. 5 components of mindful exercise - Headspace
46. Relationship between Shoulders and Hips - Susan Martin (sportsmassageearley.co.uk)
47. How to Build Awareness of the Spine - YouTube
48. Motions of the Joints of the Pelvis (sacroiliac joints) (learnmuscles.com)
49. Shoulder girdle: anatomy, movements and function | Kenhub
50. What to Expect at Pelvic Physical/Occupational Therapy - Pelvic Guru anal exam, incontinence, internal pelvic therapy, pelvic floor, pelvic global, Pelvic Guru, pelvic occupational therapy, pelvic OT, pelvic pain, pelvic physical therapy, pelvic physiotherapy, Pelvic PT, sexual dysfunction, sexual pain, starting pelvic therapy, vaginal exam, what to expect
51. Abdominal Bracing | The small nuance that makes a big difference (muscleandmotion.com)
52. Abdominal Bracing | Strength for Women | Personal Trainer New Malden (rachellawfitness.com)
53. Back Muscles: Anatomy and Function of Upper, Middle & Lower Back (clevelandclinic.org)
54. Diaphragmatic Breathing and Its Benefits (healthline.com)
55. Tips for Pelvic Floor Relaxation - Pelvic Guru hip openers, how do i get my pelvic floor to relax, how do i stretch my pelvic floor, hyptertonic pelvic floor, overactive pelvic floor, pelvic floor, pelvic floor physiotherapy, pelvic floor relaxation, pelvic floor therapy, pelvic global, pelvic global academy, Pelvic Guru, Pelvic Guru Academy, pelvic OT, pelvic physical therapist, pelvic physical therapy, pelvic physiotherapy, Pelvic PT, relaxation, stretches for pelvic floor

CH 7
56. The ideal stretching routine - Harvard Health

CH 8
57. How to add core exercises to your workout routine - Harvard Health
58. What Muscles Do Planks Work? (healthline.com)

CH 12
59. Older Adult Falls Data | Fall Prevention | Injury Center | CDC
60. Facts About Falls | Fall Prevention | Injury Center | CDC
61. Can You Die From Loneliness? | Psychology Today
62. Falls (who.int)
63. Facts About Falls | Fall Prevention | Injury Center | CDC
64. About falls risk factors - Stay On Your Feet | Queensland Health
65. Don't be the fall guy - Harvard Health

135